The Anabolic Index:

Optimized Nutrition and Supplementation Manual

David Barr

Credits

Co-Editors: David S. Lounsbury M.Sc. (Exercise Sciences)
Jeffrey D. Urdank

Associate Editor: Sabrina A. Barr

Graphic Designer: Kevin Worley

Published by F.Lepine Publishing
ISBN 978-0-9809415-2-4

Disclaimer

The contents of this manual are to be viewed as examples of nutritional and supplementation practices. The information represents a synthesis of a large volume of research, but the interpretation should be viewed as learned opinion from someone who lives and breathes fitness and nutrition, and continually strives for physical and mental greatness. What it is not, however, is a prescription. These protocols are intended for use by healthy individuals, after due consultation with a physician. As such, the author assumes no liability for any damages or personal injury acquired as a result of acting on any of the information contained herein, including but not limited to: physical or mental impairment, lost productivity, failed drug screens, litigation (some supplements might be illegal in certain locales), or death.

Conflicts of Interest: None.

The author has no financial interest in any nutritional supplement and is not affiliated with any related company.

4

TABLE OF CONTENTS

ONE

Preface

"They could be made to accept the most flagrant violations of reality, because they never fully grasped the enormity of what was demanded of them, and were not sufficiently interested in public events to notice what was happening. … They simply swallowed everything…"
-George Orwell, 1984

Knowledge Acquisition: The Most Important Section

"I know."
-Han Solo, Episode V

While driving home from the gym with my training partner Kevin, the subject of North Korea came up. During the course of discussion I mentioned Seoul (South Korea) and how I'd recently read that it is now the most populous city in the world. Without hesitation, Kevin informed me that I was wrong and proceeded to list off the "real" cities that met the criterion of 'most populated'.

I was struck by the fact that he had immediately dismissed what I had read in favor of what he had read. No information was weighed at all. He didn't question my source, explain his, or explore the semantics of what comprised a "city". Irrelevant all, he was right and I was wrong. He had made the mistake of taking his acquired information and passing it off as his own, while similarly taking the information from my source and labeling it as mine. Suddenly what we had read had become our own opinions, and the battle lines were drawn.

Now if he had been conducting research on this topic and could quote World Health Organization data, that would be one thing, but this was just two guys talking smack after a leg workout. He had read something and so did I, there was no additional research performed to see which data set was more reflective of reality.

Stated plainly, we had both come across information, but somehow he had come to believe his to the exclusion of other possibilities, without any real justification for doing so ('human nature' is an excuse, not a justification). This is a dangerous situation to be in because it not only hinders learning, but also serves to propagate incorrect information.

We are living in the Information Age, with practically unlimited information available to us. The way in which we acquire, analyze, and disseminate this information is of critical importance, now more than ever. If we can begin to consider our sources, and understand the difference between subjectivity and objectivity then we'll be much better off.

Weighing Information

The point of all of this is that there will undoubtedly be data presented in this manual that contradict traditionally held beliefs. Rather than outright rejecting this novel information because it differs from what we previously believed, or what we want to believe (as we so often do), it is critical that we weigh all of the information for its value and proceed from there.

For example:

1) What does the source that is presenting the information have to gain from the presentation of these specific data?

2) What is the track record of the information source? Have they written numerous objective and innovative rock-solid articles on the topic, or do they have a track record for blatantly lying?

3) What is their supporting evidence? Do they have any? [NOTE: This gets tricky because it has become standard practice to present only the data that support one's point of view, or reference data that are not from qualified sources]

4) It is also important to question our own motivation, because hey, we're human and we have biases. If we can recognize the opinion for which we have a greater desire to believe, then this can be incorporated into the whole of objectively weighing information.

Although this section provides information that may go beyond traditional contents of a muscle building book, the beauty is that this is the one section that can be applied in every aspect of one's life (hence the title: The Most Important Section).

Quick Tip: The internal conflict between a previously held opinion and contrary evidence is called cognitive dissonance, and often manifests itself in anger. Once we get past this stage we are more likely to be objective –but even then, weighing information is a process, not an event.

[If you're interested, sources list Seoul as the most populous city, but ONLY when counting inhabitants within actual city limits, which seems misrepresentative of a true population.]

A Short (But Important) Note About Statistics

'There are three kinds of lies: lies, damned lies, and statistics."
-Benjamin Disraeli

Most of us are familiar with statistics as they are applied in every day use. For example: "3 out of 4 people love chocolate" or "92% of Anabolic Index readers have an IQ >120". But when it comes to scientific studies, we see statistics as the mathematical science used to analyze data.

Why Should You Care?

Quite simply because this is the basis for how all scientific information is determined valid or invalid. It's simply a matter of numbers and subsequent analysis.

In order to determine that the result of a study is true, the statistical analyses must show that the results are 95% likely to be due to the intervention, rather than just chance. For example, let's say that we are trying to see whether supplement X has a real impact on muscle growth. One group will use the supplement in question (Group A) and the other (Group B) will use a placebo (inert substance).

By the end of the study group A gained an average of 3 pounds more than group B. Sounds pretty good, but are the results deemed statistically significant? Stated differently; can it be mathematically determined that the difference in results is less than 5% likely to be due to random chance? (That's a mouthful!) If the answer is no, then the results will be deemed invalid despite the average growth increase of 3 pounds!

What if we only had 1 person in each group? Then it's far more likely that random chance played a role in the results, because genetic responses between different people can be quite large. Now what if we had 1000 people in each group and we still saw an average of a 3 pound muscle difference? Then the results are far more likely to be due to the supplement, because genetic (and environmental) differences would have weeded themselves out with such large groups.

The point of all of this is that even with the utmost care and respect for the studies, there still remains an element of subjectivity when interpreting scientific data. This is why studies must always be analyzed with caution, and dogma completely avoided. Some people live and die by the 95% rule, thereby missing out on potentially advantageous research. Still others are far too lax and simply believe anything without any kind of stringent guidelines.

It's important to bear all of this in mind when analyzing any kind of information.

Quick Tip: Stats suck. (But they're a necessary evil.)

TWO

Introduction

"I think we ought always to entertain our opinions with some measure of doubt. I shouldn't wish people dogmatically to believe any philosophy, not even mine."
-Bertrand Russell

Getting the Most Out of This Manual

At first this may seem like a silly section because most instruction manuals are written with the expectation that readers will follow it in its entirety, without variation. But if there's one important lesson I've learned over the years of working with people, it's that no one program works for everyone. This is of course due to genetic differences, but more importantly for our purposes the psychological differences are key.

For example, the majority of my clients would benefit from performing squats –in effect this could be considered the ideal exercise. But the problem is that most clients absolutely despise doing them. While my old philosophy would have required them to "suck it up" and do what I thought was best for them, experience has taught that this kind of rigidity helps no one.

In fact, in these early days of my training dogma, I quickly found that when I wasn't around, many clients started substituting other exercises for squats. Some ended up going to other trainers who could help them have fun while training, while others ended up quitting altogether. All of this because I felt that because I was hardcore, others had to do what I did. I wasn't hardcore, I was dogmatic, and it took me some time to see that people are better off doing something, even if it's not exactly optimal, rather than quitting because I forced them to do something they really didn't like.

How This Applies

The point of all of this is that there should be no "must do's" in this manual. Although the contents contain an idealized plan for muscle growth and recovery, it is not expected that everyone follow every suggestion to the letter –and certainly not all at once. It is critical that you decide what you like and use it. Now I fully encourage you to consider everything, but only keep what you like and discard the rest (at least temporarily) –this rather than the alternative of ignoring the entire plan because there is a part or two that doesn't suit your preferences.

Take your time and have fun with it. You have all the time in the world to play around and experiment. If you like something then great! But if not, then file it away and maybe try it again a month or a year later. There is no time limit. Then pick up the next section that you want to try and go for it!

The Man Who Saved the World

"It is better to deserve honors and not have them than to have them and not deserve them."
--Mark Twain

Some of you may know me as the guy who worked for NASA. Some will know me as a sports supplement expert. Others will know me as a strength coach, while others still will have no idea who I am. Well, to set the record straight, I'm going to tell you who I am: as the subheading indicates, I am the man who saved the world. At least that's how I thought I was going to be perceived, but my cockeyed optimism and unbridled enthusiasm may have been a little premature.

It really began with my first objective scientific review on the amino acid glutamine. In this review article, I debunked the myth of supplementing with glutamine for athletic or physique enhancement, and to my knowledge was the first person to thoroughly do so. Of course I imagined that this would lead to fame, fortune, and an endless stream of "thank you's" from adoring fans who saved hundreds of dollars because of my work. Hell, ticker tape parades were not out of the question!

Harsh Reality

In reality, what I received were a few angry letters from people who didn't want to deal with reality, and a big bull's-eye on my forehead from the supplement industry, who had to scramble to convince their legions of followers that I was wrong (sadly, a task all too easily accomplished in the absence of any reason or evidence). Forget the parade, I barely even garnered a "thanks". Undeterred, I went on to the next bit of work, and this time, I was sure to change the world.

Instead of treading upon ingrained dogma and showing people what *didn't* work, I was going to be positive and show people what *did* work. What's more, I was going to back it up with direct scientific evidence, not theories or guesses. The best part was that I was going to take the holy grail of sports nutrition and *improve* upon it!

To be more specific, I was going to show people how they could <u>double</u> their muscle growth and recovery response to a post workout meal!

Okay, in reality, this scientifically supported idea wasn't going to change the world, but to me, this area of applied research *was* my entire world, and the implications were staggering. So when I presented the data, along with how to apply it and several other nifty scientific tidbits, I was a little surprised by the reaction –or rather, *lack of* reaction. It wasn't really negative, but then again it wasn't really much of anything at all. Words like "neat" "swell" and "hey I'm hungry" were the general lackluster replies to this information.

Rethinking Power

So I went back to the drawing board. I realized that clearly this information was too powerful for people to pass up; the problem had to be with my delivery. In other words, people just didn't understand what I was really trying to say. That's fine, science is a difficult language, and this particular area of nutritional biochemistry can give even a PhD a run for his/her money. I repackaged the information, added a whole bunch of other tricks to improve the muscle growth and recovery response and threw it out for the public to feast on. The result? Nothing. No distain, merely apathy.

This is when I knew that something was seriously wrong. Not only had I shown the ground breaking research in a different way, I had added new tricks that should have had people beating down my door to thank me.

A Beating of a Different Sort

Okay, I'm being melodramatic here. I'm not a megalomaniac and I never expected fame, fortune, or "fans" just for writing a couple of articles. But considering the amount of time and effort people are putting into achieving their goals, and the money they waste on bogus supplements, I really did think that there would be more of a positive reaction towards directly scientifically supported information. I mean, everyone believes that post-workout meals are fundamental for helping you achieve your goals, so if I can show how to make this cornerstone even better, then there would be some kind of positive reaction.

While the message has reached many people, and it is well established that pre-workout meals can have a superior effect to those consumed afterwards (as good as post-workout meals are), the difficulty in translating the cryptic language of science into clearly understandable and applicable terms remains incredibly challenging. Considering the wealth of vital information available, there had to be an easier way.

Enter The Anabolic Index

The Anabolic Index is a simple quantification of the effect that a certain supplement, drug, or dietary practice can have on muscle growth and recovery. In other words, a number is slapped on to things to show how they affect our body, much like a score. For example, something that has a very powerful impact on muscle will receive a high number, while something with a small impact will receive a low number or even zero. There are even things that can hinder muscle growth and recovery, and they are given a negative number.

The ultimate goal of this manual is to not only show you what the best practices are, how much they are better than another practice etc., but also to show you how to minimize the negative effectors, to ensure that you are using the highest Anabolic Index Score possible, and subsequently the greatest results. By maximizing your Anabolic Potential, you will notice increases in muscle growth, recovery, and performance.

Time to get started.

How Is The Anabolic Index Score Determined?

"The important thing is not to stop questioning. Curiosity has its own reason for existing."
-Albert Einstein

In order to derive scores for The Anabolic Index, the scientific literature is analyzed and directly applied. For example, scientific data showing accrued lean body mass are used to formulate the numbers. This objective derivation ensures that subjective opinions, like those on the bodybuilding message boards, or those heard around the gym, are largely (but not always) ignored. Stated more plainly, this means that opinions from guys like Johnny Bravo (a.k.a. Muscle_Blasta72), who "know" that their vitamin and mineral 'stack' gets them 'jacked and swole', have little place here.

That is not to say that subjective opinions are completely ignored, but their value is always weighed against that of hard data (See The Placebo Effect for more information). In fact, first hand data from numerous clients and athletes is also used to provide the "fine tuning" that is required to make the most accurate assessments possible.

There should be no dogma accepted from the scientific literature, but the controlled environments in which studies are conducted provide objective information that is far more reliable than that which can be experienced subjectively by a single individual.

What About the Supplements?

For too long we have been victims of the supplement industry whose goal it is to sell product at all costs. Never before has there been an industry based on lies and false promises whose all-too-eager "victims" forget the failures and beg for the next golden calf.

Think about it; we've been promised for decades that we'll have super muscle builders, but what do we have that has withstood time and testimony? Creatine and protein powders. This after literally dozens, if not hundreds of products, have been thrown at us. With such a dismal success rate, how is it that the supplement industry is now bigger than ever?

If the American auto industry had a 2% success rate, which is about where the supplement industry track record lies, the American economy would be on the verge of collapse and there would be rioting in the streets. Absolutely no one would buy these cars. You'd have to be crazy to!

But here we are with the supplement industry thriving more than ever. Despite being burned, many people still believe the lies without question, and no one calls out the companies for their deceit. Even most writers, who sell the vast majority of supplements through their articles, do nothing because the magazines they write for sell either advertising or products. It is a vicious cycle that can only end when enough people take a stand.

The benefits of such action have already been seen when, due to popular "request", the makers of a popular protein supplement opted to remove the potentially harmful ingredient "Crea-Toxin" (glycocyamine) from their product. It is just the beginning.

In reading this manual you are taking the first step of personal responsibility by taking time to learn about what you might be putting in your body.

Case Study: Us

It is absolutely amazing that we (myself included) can develop an emotional attachment to the idea that a particular supplement or technique works. If someone comes along and presents hard data to show that our beloved item doesn't work the way we would have hoped, it is natural to feel a little uneasy and resist this new information. It's human nature (recall cognitive dissonance).

The elegance of The Anabolic Index lies not only in the simplicity of the scoring system, but also in the fact that it is both fluid and objective.

That is to say that although the general ideas of The Anabolic Index are solid, the specific numbers are undergoing continual refinement. This type of adaptation and absolute lack of dogma is critical in developing a long-lasting standard by which products and practices are evaluated.

Also paramount are the objective means through which The Anabolic Index Scores are derived. By thoroughly reviewing the scientific literature and measured responses, and by scrutinizing subjective opinions, we eliminate much of the guesswork and hearsay associated with our inherently subjective opinions. And since there is no dogma here, the real beauty is that you're encouraged to form your own opinions.

For example, our friend Johnny Bravo (a 16 year old with 1 month of training experience) doesn't agree with the overwhelming evidence that plant sterols have no real impact on muscle growth. That's fine, he doesn't have to! This Manual simply presents the available evidence -it isn't trying to convince you of anything.

Conceptual Focus

Although it can be easy to get engrossed by the numbers of The Anabolic Index Score, I cannot emphasize enough that it is the underlying <u>concepts</u> that should remain the focus. The numbers are simply to serve as a quantitative guide -an easy to follow reference from which the concepts can be better applied.

THREE

Important Basics

This section largely contains the information you'd find in any other nutrition book. As the title indicates, it may be basic for some, yet is essential to understanding the fundamentals of how food can work for you, and the basis for The Anabolic Index.

Calories And Nutrients

What *is* a Calorie Anyway?

A Calorie is simply a unit of energy that we use when discussing food intake. For example, if you've eaten 3000 Calories today, you have simply added 3000 of these energy units to your body. Our body uses this energy for any of the billions of processes that are occurring in you right now. Exercise "burns Calories", which means that it takes energy to get our body moving, and the energy units are used to quantify the amount of energy expended. Generally speaking, if we take in more energy than we use up, our body can store it (as body fat and muscle), or simply burn it off as heat (which happens in people who eat anything but just can't get fat).

Calories exist in the form of food —more specifically the macronutrients: fats, carbohydrates, and proteins. For the most part, it is the latter nutrient that is the focus for The Anabolic Index, although later in the manual, the role that carbohydrates and fats play in muscle growth will be discussed.

Quick Tip: Only the macronutrients yield Caloric energy. Quantitatively they provide 4, 4, and 9 Calories per gram for Protein, Carbohydrates, and Fats. Alcohol yields 7 Calories per gram, but no, it isn't a nutrient.

Carbohydrates

This macronutrient, also known as "carbs" or "CHO"[*], is our primary source of energy that we derive from food. Types of carbohydrates include starches, sugars, and fiber.

In The Anabolic Index, focus on this nutrient for glycogen storage is only marginally important, relative to that of protein. This is not because carbohydrates are unimportant for post-training and event recovery, but rather that they are an integral part of assisting our ingested protein to optimize our results. In other words, by focusing on maximizing the positive effect of protein, we will undoubtedly maximize our glycogen storage without necessitating any focus.

[*]Due to the chemical make up of all carbohydrates: Carbon, Hydrogen, and Oxygen, respectively.

Fats

Also known as lipids, this nutrient has gotten a bad rap over the past couple of decades due to its high Caloric density. This means that compared to CHO and protein, fats yield more than twice the Calories per gram. They are found in every food, especially meat and nut products, but in their purest form they are oils.

Ingested fats are used for insulation of our organs and nerve cells, stored as energy reserves (i.e. bodyfat), and they make up a large proportion of our cell membranes. A practical discussion of how to use this nutrient is found later in the manual.

Amino Acids and Protein

Throughout the manual, the terms amino acids and protein are used continuously, but what the heck are they? Protein is a macronutrient, largely derived from animal sources, that helps with building and repair of body tissues. Different protein sources can contain different types of protein molecules or proteins (for example, the two main proteins in milk are called whey and casein), but they're all pretty much broken down to the same thing; amino acids. If a protein is like a house, then amino acids are like the bricks that build the house. Stated another way; they are the tiny molecules that make up a protein.

NOTE: For the sake of simplicity, amino acids and protein will be used interchangeably (unless otherwise specified).

Essential Digestion

Now the whole point of protein digestion is to take a protein source (like a hamburger) and break it down into its component parts (the amino acids). This process is largely accomplished in the small intestine, which is also where the amino acids are subsequently absorbed to enter the bloodstream. Once there, our body then uses these amino acids to make the different proteins our body needs.

For example, if we cause micro-damage to our biceps during a workout (which is actually the main goal of a muscle-building routine), our body will sense this, and then signal the biceps to take the amino acids from the blood in order to repair the damaged muscle –even make it bigger and stronger to resist future damage.

To summarize the process:

1) Eat Protein
2) Protein is broken down into amino acids
3) Amino acids are absorbed into the bloodstream
4) Amino acids are used by the various tissues of the body

The Anabolic Index: How This Relates

To get more specific about The Anabolic Index, we will focus in on the discussion of damaged muscle repair. To reiterate, this muscle damage acts as a signal for amino acids to be taken up, from the blood, by the muscle cells, so they can make new proteins. Of course these new proteins are built not only to repair the damaged tissue, but to build it up bigger and stronger than before; this process is known as protein synthesis and is part of the basis for The Anabolic Index.

NOTE: Muscle growth, repair, and recovery are all related to protein synthesis, and for our purposes will be used interchangeably (unless otherwise specified).

Key Point: Protein Synthesis is the Universal Goal

If you're reading this manual, then you're interested in stimulating protein synthesis (even if you didn't know it). Every time you hit the gym, the track, or the field you are stimulating protein synthesis -because it doesn't just happen with muscle, it happens with our nerve cells as well! So even if you're training for just strength or speed, you're after protein synthesis. Interestingly, if fat loss is your goal, you need to stimulate protein synthesis in order to hang on to muscle tissue as our body tries to slow down the amount of energy used.

Anabolism: Protein Synthesis

Most of us know that the most common way to stimulate protein synthesis is to hit the gym, but this is just one way. Another stimulator of muscle repair and recovery is through anabolic hormones. Hormones are just signaling molecules secreted into our blood, and we all have a dozen of them circulating all of the time. Testosterone, insulin, growth hormone, and IGF-1 are known as the anabolic hormones, because they all stimulate growth and repair of body tissues. The term anabolic simply refers to an energy consuming metabolic process (e.g. building muscle).

NOTE: For our purposes the term protein synthesis refers specifically to that process occurring in skeletal muscle, not other tissues.

Although anabolic hormones can have a large impact on muscle size and strength, high levels are needed for prolonged periods of time. Attempting to acutely stimulate (or "spike") an anabolic hormone likely has little impact on performance and growth. Of course using external sources of hormones (such as anabolic steroids) is a completely different situation altogether, as this process utilizes relatively high concentrations of the substance over a prolonged period.

Necessary Components

To further illustrate the role of hormones, it should be noted that stretched and trained muscle can stimulate protein synthesis even in the complete absence of anabolic hormones. This is because training itself is a stimulator of muscle growth and repair. Of course elevating the anabolic hormones can help us achieve our goals and is quite desirable, although this should not be our main focus. This is because we know that our ability to intentionally manipulate our hormones is rather limited compared to what we can accomplish by optimizing our biochemistry through nutrition.

Key Point: Acute hormonal manipulation has limited functionality due to our body's resistance to such changes. Although this was a great idea more than a decade ago, we have moved into the age of nutritional biochemistry –a far more effective method for optimization.

The Building Analogy

In order to understand the process of muscle growth and repair, we need only look at a construction site to see all of the players involved. Building a muscle really is a lot like building a house; we need building materials, a foreman to get the work going and workers to carry out the job. Remember that the goal is to build a bigger and stronger muscle.

Needs:

1. **Building Materials**
2. **Foreman and Workers**

If we're going to use something to represent building materials for muscle, it's clear that protein is the material that fits here. Practically speaking, we know that it's important to get enough protein in our diet to supply our body with the building materials it needs for growth and repair (See the FAQ I Section entitled: "How Much Protein Do We Need?" for more information). If you'll recall from the section on digestion, our body breaks it down and ultimately uses it to make new body proteins (among other things).

How do we get the start (and finish) signals for building and recovery? The obvious answer here is resistance training. By training the muscle we stress our body, which in turn responds by making the muscle bigger and stronger.

Putting this together we have:

1. **Building Materials = Protein**
2. **Foreman and Workers = Resistance Training**

An argument could be made that hormones also apply here, although they help muscle growth to proceed, rather than stimulate it directly. This means that in the absence of a resistance training stimulus, anabolic hormones are largely ineffectual.

NOTE: The effects of endogenous hormonal manipulation, which is what is being discussed, differs tremendously from exogenous hormone administration.

Old Thinking

This analogy may be simple and seem helpful, but for our purposes it is antiquated. The updated thinking on which The Anabolic Index is based states that nutritional intervention can optimize our biochemistry such that there is another stimulus for Anabolism, and this is but the first **Key** to The Anabolic Index.

Catabolism: Protein Breakdown

Before we get to the Keys of The Anabolic Index, a brief explanation of Catabolism is needed. I can assure you that once we get going, things are going to fly fast, and this discussion will help a great deal.

Hitting The Catabolic Wall

We're off to a good start if we're optimizing anabolism, but we're not quite at our maximum potential for growth and recovery. If we're only looking at anabolism then we're missing half of the equation, and as a result we would be missing half of our Anabolic Potential. As you might know, the Yin to the Yang of anabolism is muscle breakdown a.k.a. Catabolism. By understanding how to both maximize anabolism and minimize catabolism we'll be sure to optimize our results.

In order to fully wrap our heads around the whole anabolic/catabolic issue, let's use an analogy of building a wall. Our goal is to build the longest wall possible, as fast as we can. The catch is that there are people whose goal is to constantly tear down the wall in order to scavenge the valuable building materials. Under normal circumstances, the guys build up the wall just as fast as those breaking it down, so there's no change in overall length.

It stands to reason that if we want to extend the wall then we can simply increase the rate at which it's being built. This will certainly accomplish the basic task of making the wall longer, but there's another way to look at the problem. Even if we didn't increase the rate at which the builders work, we can still extend the wall by slowing down the guys who tear it down!

A Mongolian Example

Let's look at a specific example. Let's say that the builders who add on to the wall throw on 10 feet per day, and the other group breaks it down at 10 feet per day. If these rates were unchanged then there would be no changes in wall length because 10 feet added minus 10 feet removed equals zero feet gained. Now if we increase the rate of building to 15 feet per day then we'll add an extra 5 feet every day. Similarly, if we maintain the original rate of 10 feet added per day but then decreased the breakdown by 5 feet, then we'll also have a net gain of 5 feet per day (10 feet added - 5 feet broken down = 5 feet added).

Going back to the original plan you may recall that the goal isn't just to increase wall length, but to do it maximally and as quickly as possible. This can be accomplished by not only increasing the rate at which the wall is built, but also decreasing the breakdown. Using the same numbers as before: 15 feet added each day - 5 feet broken down =10 feet added. Clearly this combination of practices is the optimal way of achieving our goals as quickly as possible.

The processes in this wall analogy are not unlike those of muscle, which is constantly undergoing breakdown and build up. Resistance training greatly increases the rate of both muscle breakdown and build up, but the latter to a greater extent such that muscle actually grows -if the conditions are right.

Sex and Breakdown

There's no doubt that you've already heard of increasing muscle growth by stimulating anabolism, but why has the catabolic part of the equation been almost completely ignored.

1) Intuition. When we want to build something up it only makes sense to add more to it. The idea of hindering breakdown just doesn't immediately come to mind.

2) Not Sexy. Increasing anabolism is positive, easily conceivable, and just plain sexy. Anticatabolism is none of the above.

3) Too Few/Too Easy. Compared to stimulating anabolism, there are relatively few ways to decrease muscle breakdown (despite what you'll read in a bodybuilding magazine). Additionally, it's almost too easy to do, and for some reason, complicated methods/techniques lend more to sex appeal.

In spite of all of this, it is important to realize that anticatabolism is just as important as anabolism when it comes to maximizing muscle growth and recovery. This is why we have **Key #3** in The Anabolic Index.

Key Point: Eliminating catabolism is just as important as optimizing anabolism, but so far we simply have more ways of manipulating the latter.

32

FOUR

The Protein FAQ I

"Facts change, but my opinion never does."
-Stephen Colbert

1. How Much Protein Do We Need?

The implications of the answer to this one question are so great that is requires an entire section devoted to it –because it is the answer to this question that has been holding everyone back for so long, and this is the updated conclusions that will make all the difference.

The question has been kicked around for decades, but for the most part, the answer has yet to evolve from the 80's. The common bodybuilding dogma dictates that one gram of protein per pound of bodyweight be consumed each day for optimum muscle growth. In contrast, traditional scientific dogma states that only 0.8g/kg be consumed each day for the average person–which is nearly *one third* of the other recommendation!

Clearly the suggestions are mutually exclusive, so how can each exist? More importantly, how can each exist with such fervor behind them? Well, both camps have their sets of evidence: the bodybuilders have a lot of BIG men to back up their claim, while researchers have numerous studies (and big brains) to back up theirs.

Brain Washing: A Two-Way Street

The clash of these ideas came to full bear on me when I attended a talk given by the (then) worlds' expert on muscle growth and resistance training. I was incredibly excited to meet him, because coming from a bodybuilding background, it was his research that I first began to read. What's more, he was a friend of my academic advisor, so I was sure to get a chance to speak with him and learn the untold "secrets" of hypertrophy.

But something was off during his presentation. Not only did he not reveal anything new about hypertrophy training, he seemed dead set against the entire industry (a position that would take me a while to understand). To illustrate this point he focused on bodybuilders and their exorbitant protein intakes. To this day, I remember his slide containing the picture of the brain being scrubbed –his clever interpretation of brain washing. While this was somewhat amusing and got a rise out of the crowd, I was completely offended. After all, *I* was one of the people he was talking about! *I* was one of the people who bought into the dogma of the bodybuilding magazines! But *I* was also the biggest guy in the room. Hmmm...

The Old Answer

So how much protein do we, as active resistance training individuals, really need? Without getting into all of the irrelevant data, it seemed clear that consuming 1.7g of protein per kg of bodyweight (0.8g/lb) is perfectly adequate for muscle growth. In fact, the most often referenced study shows that consuming 1.4g/kg provided the same benefit as 2.4g/kg. This research supports lower values than you might expect because it used trained athletes (which is more applicable to most of us), whereas most others use untrained individuals.

Untrained people are very bad at handling protein, and subsequently have a greater need for it due to the novelty of the resistance training stimulus. Once our bodies get used to training, our biochemistry becomes more efficient at dealing with protein intake, not to mention the fact that we induce less stress during training -so ultimately we need less protein when trained.

Old Question. Old Answer

None of this information has ever sat well with bodybuilders. In fact, there seems to be the general feeling that there's a scientific conspiracy to reduce overall protein intake so that everyone looks like an endurance athlete. This may be because, bodybuilders tend to be very set in their ways, dogmatic if you will, and resistant to ideas that we don't like -even in the face of evidence to the contrary. Hell, I see this every time I present a supplement review.

So if you don't like the answer then maybe we're asking the wrong question. Perhaps then, it might be better to start asking what is *optimal*?

New Question. New Answer

So if we then ask the new question as "How much protein is optimal?", we will get a very different answer. This is because protein should not be looked at solely from a standpoint of muscle growth, but rather overall performance and body composition.

This means that although traditional protein studies simply looked at muscle building, there are other benefits to consuming high protein diets. For example, when consumed in excess, protein is the macronutrient least likely to be deposited as bodyfat. That is not to say that you can't get fat from it, but it is certainly far less likely than when overconsuming carbs or fat.

Additionally, protein consumption results in a relatively high rate of energy utilization for digestion. This means that the body burns more Calories when protein is ingested, compared to carbs and fats. Once again, the advantages of protein overconsumption at the avoidance of bodyfat are obvious. We will see elsewhere in this manual that Caloric excess is required for optimal muscle growth, it seems that protein is the nutrient of choice.

Although there are several advantages to protein overconsumption, there is one side effect. Fortunately you will be shown how to treat it.

Excess Protein: The Down Side

Higher protein intakes cause more protein to be burned off in trained athletes without increasing protein utilization (or storage) in muscle. This means that consuming "too much" protein would be seen as a mild stress by our body, which then takes steps to increase the amount of protein burned off and excreted. This type of regulatory mechanism happens with most things in our body in order to maintain balance a.k.a. homeostasis. The good news is that we can deal with it, and the prevention of this side effect is **Key #3** of The Anabolic Index.

Quick Tip: We've found over the past few years that athletes need fewer carbohydrates than once thought, and can perform optimally on higher protein diets.

The Next Level

Now that we've gone through all of the information and asked the right question, the playing field has changed once again –but don't worry, it is a very good thing.

Seemingly out of nowhere, one relatively unknown study showed that supplementing with protein actually helped to build muscle. You may not have heard about it because it is often labeled and read as a creatine study, otherwise the supplement companies would have been all over it.

As if to prove that it wasn't a fluke, a series of recent studies have all come out to demonstrate that increased protein intakes result in improved muscle growth. But if the story was settled 15 years ago, what accounts for the renewed surge in data? In short; whey protein.

This information is exciting enough that is was developed into **Key #4** of The Anabolic Index.

Quick Tip: It seems as though Caloric excess, regardless of which nutrient it comes from, is more important than overall protein intake in training novices. So if you fall into this category, concern yourself with Calories, not just protein.

Practical Application

With all of this novel information, we need to figure out how to put it together in order to achieve our goals. This is done in the following sections, and wrapped up in the "Putting It All Together" section.

Selected References

Position of the American Dietetic Association, Dietitians of Canada, and the American College of Sports Medicine: Nutrition and athletic performance. J Am Diet Assoc. 2000 Dec;100(12):1543-56

Burke DG, Chilibeck PD, Davidson KS, Candow DG, Farthing J, Smith-Palmer T.
The effect of whey protein supplementation with and without creatine monohydrate combined with resistance training on lean tissue mass and muscle strength. Int J Sport Nutr Exerc Metab. 2001 Sep;11(3):349-64

Fielding RA, Parkington J. What are the dietary protein requirements of physically active individuals? New evidence on the effects of exercise on protein utilization during post-exercise recovery. Nutr Clin Care. 2002 Jul-Aug;5(4):191-6

Lemon PW. Protein and amino acid needs of the strength athlete. Int J Sport Nutr. 1991 Jun;1(2):127-45 Sports Med. 1991 Nov;12(5):313-25

Lemon PW, Proctor DN. Protein intake and athletic performance.

Phillips SM. Protein requirements and supplementation in strength sports. Nutrition. 2004 Jul-Aug;20(7-8):689-95

Phillips SM, Hartman JW, Wilkinson SB. Dietary protein to support anabolism with resistance exercise in young men. J Am Coll Nutr. 2005 Apr;24(2):134S-139S

Phillips SM. Dietary protein for athletes: from requirements to metabolic advantage. Appl Physiol Nutr Metab. 2006 Dec;31(6):647-54

Tipton KD, Wolfe RR. Protein and amino acids for athletes. J Sports Sci. 2004 Jan;22(1):65-79

Tipton KD, Witard OC Protein requirements and recommendations for athletes: relevance of ivory tower arguments for practical recommendations. Clin Sports Med. 2007 Jan;26(1):17-36

2. Protein: How Safe is It?

"If my answers frighten you then you should cease asking scary questions."
-Jules Winfield, Pulp Fiction

One of the most frequently debated topics among strength athletes, coaches, nutritionists, and even parents, the answers to this question have become muddled and confusing. Although no dogma should ever be accepted, we need a clear evaluation of the science and subsequent answer that we can all use.

Protein: Not as Safe as You Would Hope

Did you know that high protein diets can be harmful to more than 10% of people who use them? Yeah, I was surprised too, but if we can get the word out we can do something about it.

For the most part protein consumption doesn't seem to be inherently harmful to the majority of the population. The problem lies in those with even mild kidney dysfunction (a.k.a. renal dysfunction, a.k.a. renal insufficiency). "No big deal" you say, "I don't have any problems with my kidneys." Well, maybe you do.

In fact, the real issue here is that nearly everyone with mild kidney dysfunction has no idea they even have it! It's largely asymptomatic until later in life, or after a long duration of stress -after which more damage has been done.

What Does This Mean?

This means that there are more than 10% of people reading this manual who might have problems with handling a high protein diet, and they don't know about it. Now I'm not trying to alarm everyone by saying that high protein diets will kill you, but I am trying to raise awareness that there is potential for harm if you don't rule out mild kidney dysfunction. Simple urinalysis should do the trick, but be sure to talk to your doctor for more information.

For the rest of us (yes I've been tested), research indicates that there are no problems with consuming high protein diets -at least for a few months at a time.

Increased Risk

Although I wouldn't consider the risks to be "great", subjectively speaking, we should recognize when they may be increased. For example, we know that there is increased risk for kidney stone formation in overweight men consuming high quantities of meat protein. Although the data relating kidney stones to protein intake remain largely inconclusive, the above risk factor is noteworthy. Similarly, when hundreds of women were studied, it was shown that meat protein held more risk for those with kidney dysfunction compared to dairy and vegetable proteins. Naturally, all of this is worth discussing with your doctor.

On Bodybuilders

Gym rats are notorious for their high protein intakes of even 2-3g/lb for prolonged periods of time. Unfortunately, the highest amount ever studied has been 1.3g/lb for several months, although research suggests that kidney function may actually undergo a positive adaptation to handle these high quantities (much like our muscle adapts to the stress of resistance training). Traditionally studied "high protein diets" can use protein intakes that are *half* (!) of what the typical strength athlete consumes, so as always, further research is needed before stronger safety guidelines can be given.

Finally, it is commonly believed that higher protein intakes result in a challenge to our hydration status i.e. the amount of water our body needs. Although this myth was largely debunked in a recent study, most of us could stand to drink more water, so keep chugging away (see the Review of Water for more information).

NOTE: many of you reading this manual will be supplementing with creatine, which it seems does require increased water intake.

Quick Tip: For the most part higher protein diets seem safe and have many advantages over high carbohydrate or high fat diets.

Selected References

Brandle E, Sieberth HG, Hautmann RE. Effect of chronic dietary protein intake on the renal function in healthy subjects. Eur J Clin Nutr. 1996 Nov;50(11):734-40.

Friedman AN High-protein diets: potential effects on the kidney in renal health and disease. Am J Kidney Dis. 2004 Dec;44(6):950-62

Knight EL, Stampfer MJ, Hankinson SE, Spiegelman D, Curhan GC. The impact of protein intake on renal function decline in women with normal renal function or mild renal insufficiency. Ann Intern Med. 2003 Mar 18;138(6):460-7

Martin WF, Armstrong LE, Rodriguez NR. Dietary protein intake and renal function. Nutr Metab (Lond). 2005 Sep 20;2:25.

Martin WF, Cerundolo LH, Pikosky MA, Gaine PC, Maresh CM, Armstrong LE, Bolster DR, Rodriguez NR. 2006 Effects of dietary protein intake on Indexes of hydration. J Am Diet Assoc. 2006 Apr;106(4):587-9.

Jacques R. Poortmans; Olivier Dellalieux Do Regular High Protein Diets Have Potential Health Risks on Kidney Function in Athletes? . Int J Sport Nutr. Vol. 10, Iss. 1 2000

Taylor EN, Stampfer MJ, Curhan GC. Dietary factors and the risk of incident kidney stones in men: new insights after 14 years of follow-up. J Am Soc Nephrol. 2004 Dec;15(12):3225-32

FIVE

The 5 Keys To The Anabolic Index

"Three minutes. This is it - ground zero. Would you like to say a few words to mark the occasion?"
-Tyler Durden, Fight Club

Key #1
Protein Potential

You're probably already getting enough of the building material (protein) and you're certainly training, so we have all of the pieces of the puzzle together, right? We'll maybe not, because one of the keys to The Anabolic Index is that <u>ingesting protein can *directly* stimulate protein synthesis</u>, even in the absence of resistance training.

The Return of the Analogy

Remember our muscle building/construction site analogy? In terms of this comparison, even if the resistance training foreman isn't telling our muscle to build and repair, we have another potential foreman who can come in and do that!

This means that protein can be used not only for a building material, but also as the stimulator of protein synthesis. Evolutionarily this makes a certain amount of sense because in the presence of high quantities of protein, our body would want to store this material for times when external sources of protein are lacking. What's even better is that we can't build muscle without the raw materials (even with a perfect training program) but you can build muscle with proper use of protein.

Synergistic Application

So does this mean that we can get big from sitting around and eating hamburgers all day? Well yes, if "big" means fat, but a lean and muscular "big"? No. There are a couple of reasons why; the most obvious being that eating protein, even using The Anabolic Index, is meant to work in concert with a resistance training program. In fact, that is the application of the first key to The Anabolic Index; <u>combining proper dietary intake with an appropriate training program will promote a synergistic effect between the two anabolic signals ("foremen") to optimize muscle growth and recovery</u>.

Why Eating Protein Isn't Enough

As alluded to in the previous section, there is another reason why eating large amounts of protein doesn't make you lean and muscular, despite the tendency for amino acids to stimulate protein synthesis. In fact, this is intuitive because it is well established that simply eating more protein does not equate to a greater muscle mass.

This is due to a process that we're all familiar with called Accommodation. Although the term might be new to you, the concept is not: accommodation is the process of our body becoming accustomed to something. For example, how soon after you put on a wristwatch do you fail to notice its presence? The watch is still there, still touching your skin, but our brain no longer receives or sends us signals that it's there.

Protein Resistance

Accommodation occurs with every one of our six senses, but it also happens when we continually eat protein. In this case, nutritional accommodation occurs when our body "gets used to protein" and turns off the anabolic signal. With regard to this accommodation of protein intake, it is an undesirable state known as Protein Resistance.

The bad news is that protein resistance happens every time we eat a meal of solid protein. Due to the relatively slow digestion and absorption we have a slow trickle of amino acids into the blood. This equates to an amino acid flatline – which can be thought of as the death of protein synthesis.

NOTE: protein resistance also occurs immediately following a workout, a period known as the Post-Workout Blackout, which is covered in both the Optimizing Post-Workout Nutrition section and the Anabolic Myths section.

The good news is that 1) an amino acid flatline still allows for the possibility of an anticatabolic effect (see **Key #3**), and 2) now we are aware of this limitation so we are better able work around it -and keep muscle growth going for as long as possible. In fact, we likely do so whenever we have a whey protein shake shortly after our workouts. This ingestion of a rapidly absorbable protein Pulses our (blood) amino acid levels, which tells our body to switch on the anabolic signal once again. Interestingly, it seems that as long as our body has *increasing* amino acid levels, the anabolic signal persists and protein resistance is avoided.

Quick Tip: Following the post-workout blackout, there seems to be an enhanced period of **Protein Sensitivity**, such that protein resistance and the accommodation response are hindered for a time. This means that it is a great time for building and repairing muscle.

Selected References

Bohé J, Low JF, Wolfe RR, Rennie MJ. Latency and duration of stimulation of human muscle protein synthesis during continuous infusion of amino acids. J Physiol. 2001 Apr 15;532(Pt 2):575-9

Børsheim E, Tipton KD, Wolf SE, Wolfe RR. Essential amino acids and muscle protein recovery from resistance exercise. Am J Physiol Endocrinol Metab. 2002 Oct;283(4):E648-57

Koopman R, Wagenmakers AJ, Manders RJ, Zorenc AH, Senden JM, Gorselink M, Keizer HA, van Loon LJ. Combined ingestion of protein and free leucine with carbohydrate increases postexercise muscle protein synthesis in vivo in male subjects. Am J Physiol Endocrinol Metab. 2005 Apr;288(4):E645-53

Rasmussen BB, Tipton KD, Miller SL, Wolf SE, Wolfe RR. An oral essential amino acid-carbohydrate supplement enhances muscle protein anabolism after resistance exercise. J Appl Physiol. 2000 Feb;88(2):386-92

Rennie MJ, Bohé J, Wolfe RR. Latency, duration and dose response relationships of amino acid effects on human muscle protein synthesis. J Nutr. 2002 Oct;132(10):3225S-7S

Key #2
Protein Pulse Feeding

The advanced application of Protein Potential is the second key to The Anabolic Index. By employing this technique we are able to optimize anabolism in a way that has never been used before.

Protein Peaks

We know from the previous key that we can stimulate anabolism by increasing the levels of blood amino acids. As a corollary, the faster the increase in blood amino acids, the greater the stimulation of muscle growth. This means that if we can quickly spike or Pulse our amino acids, we will optimize the hypertrophic response.

The Particular Pulsing Proteins

In order to pulse our protein levels, we need a protein that is very quickly absorbed. Dealing with too much digestion will delay entry into the gut and subsequently the blood, which will ultimately delay the growth response. This means that whey hydrolysate is ideal for the task. As explained in greater detail in the Review of Whey Protein, hydrolyzed whey is fractionated (broken down into smaller fragments) such that it is simply a collection of amino acid chains, rather than actual proteins. This means that it will be absorbed far more quickly than other types of protein.

Additionally, whey isolate, although not ideally broken up into small peptides, will suffice as a moderate speed protein to suit most of our pulsing needs. Whey isolate is more readily available and is more of a user-friendly product.

Timing

As we've been learning over the past decade, nutrient timing is critical for optimizing our biochemistry, performance, and body composition. By Protein Pulse Feeding at appropriate times, we can take full advantage of these benefits.

1) Morning

When we awaken the level of our blood amino acids will be low. This is largely inevitable, even if we have consumed a slow protein before bed. Although it is not an ideal situation to be in, we can take advantage of it by Pulsing our amino acids shortly after we wake up. In fact, it is when our blood amino acids are low that our body is even more responsive to Protein Potential and Protein Pulse Feeding.

2) Pre-Workout

Although it originally seemed counterintuitive, Protein Pulse Feeding before a workout is the most anabolic practice we know of. By pulsing our blood amino acid levels before training, we provide an anabolic stimulus that coincides with that from training. Further, the elevated muscle blood flow during training will flood our muscle with amino acids to yield a result that is even greater than normal. Finally, any insulin released during this time (from the addition of carbohydrates or BCAA's) will magnify the amplitude of this effect by increasing the amino acids entry into muscle and enhancing blood flow even further. All of those factors combine to yield a powerful synergistic effect.

3) Post-Workout

Likely the most common application of Protein Pulse Feeding, Post-Workout nutrition has become a staple of the advanced athlete. It takes advantage of the enhanced responsiveness to insulin, increased blood flow, and optimized sensitivity to amino acids that accompany this time period. Fortunately, this period lasts far longer than once thought, leaving the "Post-Workout window of Opportunity" to last for more than 24 hours. Considering the importance placed upon post-workout feeding, it is exciting to think of the implications when this Protein Sensitivity is extended for far longer than once expected.

NOTE: The period of Post-Workout Protein Sensitivity only occurs after the Post-Workout Blackout has expired. See Anabolic Myth #3 for more information.

Although it is covered elsewhere, it is worth mentioning here that a second post-workout Protein Pulse yields identical effects to that of the first. This means that rather than having simply one Post-Workout liquid meal, a second will in effect <u>double the anabolism</u> experienced during this time.

Key Point: The antiquated notion of a post-workout window is now replaced by a prolonged period of enhanced Protein Sensitivity and Carbohydrate Tolerance.

4) Nocturnally

Reserved as a technique for only the most elite athletes, nocturnal feeding is an incredibly powerful stimulator of anabolism. By waking up in the middle of the night to spike protein with a combination of whey and casein, an anabolic Protein Pulse will precede the additional anticatabolic effect from the slower protein. For many, this type of consumption disrupts sleep to the point that it is unusable, but for those who employ it without problems the reward is great.

Quick Tips:

- Protein should be the only nutrient consumed during nocturnal feedings.

- Drinking should best occur in the dark such that light does not trigger a state of greater alertness (and subsequently result in difficulty falling back to sleep).

- Finally, waking up naturally (e.g. to use the bathroom) disrupts sleep far less than setting an alarm. Drinking more liquid before sleep can help to initiate this practice (although obvious caution must be used).

Other Times

Protein Pulse Feeding can be used at any time, although the situation becomes more complicated outside of the times mentioned. For example, solid foods will greatly slow the entry of amino acids into the blood which reduces the amplitude of the pulse. Additionally, if one is already in a highly protein-fed state, then the body is more likely to simply burn off the amino acids rather than use them for hypertrophy.

Selected References

Bohé J, Low JF, Wolfe RR, Rennie MJ. Latency and duration of stimulation of human muscle protein synthesis during continuous infusion of amino acids. J Physiol. 2001 Apr 15;532(Pt 2):575-9

Børsheim E, Tipton KD, Wolf SE, Wolfe RR. Essential amino acids and muscle protein recovery from resistance exercise. Am J Physiol Endocrinol Metab. 2002 Oct;283(4):E648-57

Calbet JA, MacLean DA. Plasma glucagon and insulin responses depend on the rate of appearance of amino acids after ingestion of different protein solutions in humans. J Nutr. 2002 Aug;132(8):2174-82.
Dangin M, Boirie Y, Garcia-Rodenas C, Gachon P, Fauquant J, Callier P, Ballevre O, Beaufrere B. The digestion rate of protein is an independent regulating factor of postprandial protein retention Am J Physiol Endocrinol Metab 280: E340-E348, 2001

Hawley JA, Tipton KD, Millard-Stafford ML. Promoting training adaptations through nutritional interventions. J Sports Sci. 2006 Jul;24(7):709-21

Koopman R, Wagenmakers AJ, Manders RJ, Zorenc AH, Senden JM, Gorselink M, Keizer HA, van Loon LJ. Combined ingestion of protein and free leucine with carbohydrate increases postexercise muscle protein synthesis in vivo in male subjects. Am J Physiol Endocrinol Metab. 2005 Apr;288(4):E645-53

Rennie MJ, Bohé J, Wolfe RR. Latency, duration and dose response relationships of amino acid effects on human muscle protein synthesis. J Nutr. 2002 Oct;132(10):3225S-7S

Key #3
Protein Withdrawal

One of the most costly mistakes when trying to optimize muscle growth building is protein fasting. At first glance this may not seem like a big deal, but bodybuilders and athletes have changed our diets such that this is now a critical anabolic factor.

Not That Bad?

The initial impression given by this idea is that if we are protein fasted then we simply do not have the building materials for growth –the implication being that we are not actually growing muscle for the short period in which we are without this vital nutrient.

I have even spoken to some who do not realize that lack of protein equates to lack of growth. They had never really given it much thought, and simply feel that muscle would get its building materials from another source. The reality is that muscle is the protein store for the rest of our body, not the other way around.

Breakdown: Fasted = Faster

So if our muscle supplies the rest of our body with protein, then protein fasting describes the periods during which our body is relying on internal muscle stores of protein for its amino acids. In other words, this is when our body is breaking down muscle due to a lack of ingested protein. This harvesting of muscle happens when *any* tissue needs amino acids, and some seem to have an insatiable appetite.

In contrast to the initial idea, a protein fasted state is one of strong catabolism rather than simply a neutral absence of anabolism. Fortunately for us, resistance training helps to mitigate the rate of protein degradation, but as you're about to see, this is in direct contrast to the dramatic fasted-state catabolism that is induced by a high protein intake.

So how do we fix it? Should we just eat even more protein?

Protein Withdrawal

Somewhat ironically, it is our intentional overconsumption of protein that induces such a problematic protein fast. This is because our bodies adapt to the high levels of ingested protein by ramping up the rate at which it's broken down. This isn't a big deal because of everything that's coming in through our mouths, but it becomes a serious issue once feeding stops.

In essence, our body comes to expect high protein intake, so if we ever decrease consumption or worse yet, fast, then our body still has all of the protein breakdown machinery going full steam. And if this machinery doesn't have external protein to break down, then they will turn on our own muscle and chew it up at an accelerated rate –a state known as Protein Withdrawal.

Although there are no deleterious side effects other than elevated muscle catabolism, in principle Protein Withdrawal is analogous to withdrawal of any other drug or addiction.

As bad as the problem may be, the potential solutions are simple: **1)** Eat less protein **2)** Ensure that we never decrease protein intake.

1) Protein: Less Is More?

If we adopt the idea of eating less protein, then the catabolic machinery won't work as hard and we don't have to worry as much about times when we are protein fasted. The problem with this "solution" is that it is sub-optimal. We'll see throughout this Manual that high protein, particularly whey, is conducive to recovery and growth. So simply eating less protein is not the way to go.

2) The Best Solution

Due to the fact that we want to take advantage of all the benefits that come along with high protein intake, the best solution to avoiding Protein Withdrawal is to ensure that we are never protein fasted. This means that while we may go periods without actually feeding, we must ensure that we still have protein feeding our body. If this sounds contradictory, check out the following examples for the application of this Key.

The Practical Component

There are three times when people commonly protein fast, every single day. By sticking to the idea of remaining protein fed, we can maintain anabolism and stave off the otherwise accelerated catabolism.

1) Pre-Workout: It is common for people to starve themselves before training. This is often due to a belief in enhanced fat loss during training, while some people may feel sick to their stomach if they have food on it. Based on the power of pre-workout nutrition, it is clear that anabolism will be enhanced and breakdown decreased if we can maintain a protein fed state.

So how do we do accomplish this without hindering our workouts? Well, if you feel sick to your stomach, then you can simply have some powdered casein a couple of hours before training. This will not be felt at all during training, but will help maintain anabolism. The same procedure can be used for those focused on intra-workout fat loss, although consuming whey alone pre-workout is an even better idea.

2) Night Time: Sleeping is the most obvious time when we protein fast, and if we don't take care of the accelerated breakdown, we're putting the brakes on muscle growth. Casein pre-bed is the best way to do this, and such drinks have been outlined in detail in the section: <u>Designing the Ultimate Protein Drink</u>.

3) Waking: It is interesting to me that many people go for so long after waking before having anything to eat. Again this could be due to nausea or a belief in enhanced fat loss during fasting.

As someone who wakes up due to hunger, it was surprising for me to learn how many people cannot, or do not want, to eat when they wake up. For the majority of people, even a scoop of whey in water is well tolerated and can work wonders for muscle growth. If the lack of desire to feed is due to early-morning grogginess (something else I experience), having a pre-made shake ready to go in the fridge is a great idea. For maximum efficiency, it can even be made at the same time as the pre-bed shake.

Quick Tip: Remember that most proteins will last in the bloodstream for more than 3 hours, so be sure to take advantage of this fact in avoiding Protein Withdrawal.

Selected References

Gaine PC, Pikosky MA, Bolster DR, Martin WF, Maresh CM, Rodriguez NR. Postexercise whole-body protein turnover response to three levels of protein intake. Med Sci Sports Exerc. 2007 Mar;39(3):480-6

Hall WL, Millward DJ, Long SJ, Morgan LM. Casein and whey exert different effects on plasma amino acid profiles, gastrointestinal hormone secretion and appetite. Br J Nutr. 2003 Feb;89(2):239-48

Millward DJ. Protein and amino acid requirements of adults: current controversies. Can J Appl Physiol. 2001;26 Suppl:S130-40

Millward DJ. An adaptive metabolic demand model for protein and amino acid requirements. Br J Nutr. 2003 Aug;90(2):249-60

Millward DJ. Macronutrient intakes as determinants of dietary protein and amino acid adequacy. J Nutr. 2004 Jun;134(6 Suppl):1588S-1596S

Pacy PJ, Price GM, Halliday D, Quevedo MR, Millward DJ. Nitrogen homeostasis in man: the diurnal responses of protein synthesis and degradation and amino acid oxidation to diets with increasing protein intakes. Clin Sci (Lond). 1994 Jan;86(1):103-16.

Price GM, Halliday D, Pacy PJ, Quevedo MR, Millward DJ. Nitrogen homeostasis in man: influence of protein intake on the amplitude of diurnal cycling of body nitrogen. Clin Sci (Lond). 1994 Jan;86(1):91-102

Key #4
Protein Prioritization

In this manual we discuss the importance of timing and it's application to muscle growth, the more general factors of quantity and quality cannot be overlooked.

Quantity of Quality

As discussed in the Protein FAQ #1, having a diet that consists of more protein than needed will help to optimize body composition –and as discussed in FAQ#2 this can be done with a high degree of safety. To be more specific about mere quantity we must subsequently define the factor of quality, with reference to protein.

Quality: The Common Thread

Although many products can be considered quality protein, such as grass fed beef or fresh Atlantic salmon, these products do not quite have the impact on our muscle growth that the highest quality protein does: whey protein.

Although this supplement has a review devoted to it in the Nutrition and Supplement Optimization manual, a more general explanation of its importance is required here. Quite simply, when it comes to whey protein, the old erroneous idea that "the more protein you eat the bigger you get", seems to be *true*. <u>Within reason</u> of course.

The New Thinking

What has amazed me when poring through the protein literature is that the majority of studies show no effect of increased protein consumption on muscle growth or performance. But more recently, studies have popped up that have in fact shown a benefit to eating more than the standard 1.4g/kg. The common thread among these newer studies? Whey protein. Each and every one.

Such a powerful finding can not be ignored. While we've understood that whey protein is the highest quality known, there has been, until recently, little interest in studying its application for anything other than acute use. Now that we're looking at longer term studies, it seems that we've finally uncovered a protein that is of high enough quality that it actually works with our biochemistry to increase muscle growth.

Now if this effect simply occurs from supplementing with whey protein in general, imagine the impact when all of the Keys of The Anabolic Index are employed.

Reasoning

Although work on whey protein is still in its infancy, there are a couple of main suggestions as to why it succeeds where all other proteins have failed. Quite simply, the amino acid profile, ease of availability, and ability for manipulation provide an effect that eclipses all other supplements. Stated differently, by having such a high utilization rate by muscle, whey protein is able to stimulate anabolism that has synergistic impact with the training effect.

Practical Application

Most people are using whey protein following a workout to enhance muscle growth and recovery, and this is a good start. Morning, pre-workout, and nocturnal drinks have all been discussed elsewhere in this manual, and help to provide an ideal amount of whey. More generally speaking however, it is not unreasonable to state that consuming one-third of the protein diet as whey protein will help to optimize muscle growth and recovery.

For example, a 200lb highly trained individual may consume 240g of protein daily. If they are using the main three times for Protein Pulse Feeding, then this will account for at least 120g of whey every training day. Considering that muscle growth is often optimized by supplemental liquid meals, even a single protein drink each day (other than the waking drink) will help to meet the daily whey quota on non-training days.

Important Note: Consuming an exact amount of any nutrient each day is enough to drive anyone crazy. Just keep everything within reasonable limits and you won't burn out by having to keep track of every gram and every Calorie.

Quick Tip: Generally speaking, quality can take the place of quantity if necessary. This means that if more hydrolyzed, or isolated whey is used, the recommendation for quantity can be reduced. For example, instead of using 1/3 of the daily protein intake as whey concentrate, 1/5 may be consumed as whey hydrolysate without the need for further supplementation.

Selected References

Burke DG, Chilibeck PD, Davidson KS, Candow DG, Farthing J, Smith-Palmer T. The effect of whey protein supplementation with and without creatine monohydrate combined with resistance training on lean tissue mass and muscle strength. Int J Sport Nutr Exerc Metab. 2001 Sep;11(3):349-64

Candow DG, Burke NC, Smith-Palmer T, Burke DG. Effect of whey and soy protein supplementation combined with resistance training in young adults. Int J Sport Nutr Exerc Metab. 2006 Jun;16(3):233-44

Cribb PJ, Williams AD, Carey MF, Hayes A.The effect of whey isolate and resistance training on strength, body composition, and plasma glutamine. Int J Sport Nutr Exerc Metab. 2006 Oct;16(5):494-509

Cribb PJ, Williams AD, Stathis CG, Carey MF, Hayes A. Effects of whey isolate, creatine, and resistance training on muscle hypertrophy. Med Sci Sports Exerc. 2007 Feb;39(2):298-307

Kerksick CM, Rasmussen CJ, Lancaster SL, Magu B, Smith P, Melton C, Greenwood M, Almada AL, Earnest CP, Kreider RB. The effects of protein and amino acid supplementation on performance and training adaptations during ten weeks of resistance training. J Strength Cond Res. 2006 Aug;20(3):643-53

Tarnopolsky MA, Parise G, Yardley NJ, Ballantyne CS, Olatinji S, Phillips SM. Creatine-dextrose and protein-dextrose induce similar strength gains during training. Med Sci Sports Exerc. 2001 Dec;33(12):2044-52.

Yalcin AS. Emerging therapeutic potential of whey proteins and peptides. Curr Pharm Des. 2006;12(13):1637-43

Key #5
Protein Protection

One of the biggest killers of muscle growth is the unnecessary destruction of the protein that we ingest. This natural phenomenon, know as protein oxidation, means that instead of protein being used for muscle building, it is simply burned off. By protecting our protein from oxidative destruction we will have more available for anabolism and recovery.

The Protein Killer

You probably know of people who can eat whatever they want and not gain an ounce of fat. In fact, there's a good chance that you may be one of those people yourself, because these same people have a tremendously hard time putting on muscle as well. Although it is commonly known as a very fast metabolism, the reality is that these people have a very high nutrient oxidation rate. This means 1) that there is likely a lot of oxidative damage going on in their body 2) any nutrient, not just protein, will be quickly broken down and not used by the body.

If you'll recall the construction analogy, this means that not only are the building materials not available for growth, but neither is the fuel energy for the process. Considering that amino acids also stimulate muscle growth, oxidation kills yet another anabolic factor.

The Up Side

The good part of all this is that there is a way to combat protein and energy oxidation, and it is known as Protein Protection. This is the process of essentially shielding our ingested protein from oxidation such that it is available for the body to use. The best part is that Protein Protection can be accomplished in a variety of different ways, so if we make use of all of them we can minimize the amount of protein destroyed.

1) Nutrients

The less specific manner of Protein Protection is to use nutrients as an oxidative shield. When they are ingested together, the body will use some of its limited resources to oxidize fats and carbohydrates, which ultimately results in less protein destroyed. Stated differently; the body can only oxidize so much at once, so if we give it more things to oxidize, then less of any one thing will be broken down.

It's like a school of fish being fed upon by a larger fish (oxidation). The more fish we have in the school, the less likely any one fish is to being eaten. This shotgun approach isn't very precise, but it's effective.

2) Insulin

The more precise protein shield is the hormone insulin. It is secreted in response to carbohydrate ingestion and possesses both anabolic and anticatabolic properties -the latter of which is largely due to an ability to inhibit catabolic and oxidative enzymes. In other words, insulin will help turn off the machinery that unnecessarily breaks down our protein.

3) Calories

This one is simple; in order to maximize ingested protein efficiency, _eat more_! Again, this is based on the fact that the body can only oxidize so much, so by adding more quantity, we will have more fuel energy for the process of muscle building.

For example, if our body oxidizes 1000 Calories a day, then we will have a greater anabolic yield from consuming 4000 (4000-1000=3000) Calories than we would from consuming 3000 Calories (3000-1000=2000). The best part is that the stimulus for growth is disproportionate with the Caloric increase. In fact, this example yields a 33% increase in anabolism despite only ingesting 25% more Calories!

In Practice

The way to make use of this information is simple; _when we eat protein, we should be eating other nutrients as well_. This could be as easy as adding carbohydrates to your post workout drink (which you should be doing anyway) or adding fat to your pre-bed shake. Some people go so far as to consume their other nutrients before protein, but this is largely unnecessary.

Quick Tips:

- The BCAA's are particularly susceptible to protein oxidation, and Protein Protection should always be practiced when consuming them.

- The faster the protein, the more susceptible it is to oxidation. Take the appropriate precautions when Protein Pulse Feeding.

- Fasting is the easiest way to increase protein oxidation, so to ensure optimal anabolism, make sure that you're never fasted.

- Oxidation is the same process by which fish oil is easily destroyed, so Protein Protection is warranted with its consumption.

- The higher the blood amino acid levels, the higher the oxidation rate will be.

Selected References

Elia M, Khan K, Jennings G. Effect of mixed meal ingestion on fuel utilization in the whole body and in superficial and deep forearm tissues. Br J Nutr. 1999 May;81(5):373-81

Gibala MJ. Protein metabolism and endurance exercise. Sports Med. 2007;37(4-5):337-40

Koopman R, Wagenmakers AJ, Manders RJ, Zorenc AH, Senden JM, Gorselink M, Keizer HA, van Loon LJ. Combined ingestion of protein and free leucine with carbohydrate increases postexercise muscle protein synthesis in vivo in male subjects. Am J Physiol Endocrinol Metab. 2005 Apr;288(4):E645-53

Pacy PJ, Price GM, Halliday D, Quevedo MR, Millward DJ. Nitrogen homeostasis in man: the diurnal responses of protein synthesis and degradation and amino acid oxidation to diets with increasing protein intakes. Clin Sci (Lond). 1994 Jan;86(1):103-16.

Rasmussen BB, Tipton KD, Miller SL, Wolf SE, Wolfe RR. An oral essential amino acid-carbohydrate supplement enhances muscle protein anabolism after resistance exercise. J Appl Physiol. 2000 Feb;88(2):386-92

Tipton KD, Ferrando AA, Phillips SM, Doyle D Jr, Wolfe RR. Postexercise net protein synthesis in human muscle from orally administered amino acids. Am J Physiol. 1999 Apr;276(4 Pt 1):E628-34

SIX

Optimizing Nutritional Supplementation

Optimization of Loading Supplements

Your first question should be: "what exactly is a loading supplement?". The answer is simple and all too familiar: a loading supplement is one that is used in such a way as to gradually increase levels of that substance in the body. Creatine is the best-known example, but beta alanine also falls into this category. We initially consume these substances in larger quantities to gradually elevate our physiological levels of them in our body –essentially loading them– after which we decrease the dosage to maintain that high level.

So why do we need a section for loading supplements?

Quite simply because the most common use of these products is sub optimal, and this manual is all about optimization. General use lacks any kind of thought or scientific basis, and consequently, you're being short changed. Now I'm not talking about something as common as inducing an insulin spike with creatine (Discussed in the Review of Creatine), I'm talking about a standardized method for application to all loading supplements.

How Loading Works

It is best to think of a loading supplement as water, and our body as a barrel. Our goal, to optimize performance and body composition is to load up the barrel with as much of the water as possible. It sounds simple, but there are a few catches.

1) We can't load up too quickly.

If we add too much water to the barrel too quickly, our body will end up excreting most of it –even though the barrel is not yet full. It's like the wood of the barrel needs time to swell to become watertight, and so must be filled gradually to avoid waste. Filling up too quickly not only wastes money, but can also have unforeseen physiological consequences.

2) We can't surpass our saturation point.

Once we're fully loaded, our body is saturated and can't accept any more and will simply excrete any excess. In contrast to loading too quickly, surpassing the saturation point is analogous to overfilling the barrel and having the water spill over the top. Again, this is a waste of money and may result in a sub optimal physiologic profile.

3) There is a hole in the barrel.

As we try to load the barrel with water, it is easy to imagine that there is a small hole in the bottom which leaks water. This is analogous to the fact that our body actually "uses up" the loading supplements, particularly when we train.

Loading Phase

In order to truly understand how loading works, we'll need a simple system of quantification to work with our analogy. We'll use creatine* as water, and cups as our quantity in this example. For the sake of simplicity let's pretend for the moment that our barrel starts out empty, which equates to starting out with a body creatine level of zero. It's not completely realistic, but then again we're using a barrel to simulate a human body, so what are you going to do.

As we begin to consume supplemental creatine we're essentially filling the barrel up with water –regardless of whether we do an official "loading phase." Even supplementing with a mere 5-10g of creatine a day could equate to adding 5 cups of water per day. Of course our body uses creatine, which could equate to a leak of one cup. In this example, we're adding a net of 4 cups of water to the barrel a day (5 cups added – 1 cup leaked).

Theoretically, if the barrel holds say 40 cups of water, then we'll be full after only 10 days of loading. If we're impatient, we could try to load all 40 cups of water in a day or two. This would likely induce a mild stress on our body and result in the majority of water being excreted. In fact, we know that even during a standard loading phase most of the creatine is excreted by the body, so a slow loading process is warranted.

Loaded: Now What?

After 10 days of adding 5 cups (net gain of 4) to the barrel, it will be completely full. At this point it is said to have reached **saturation**. This means that we just can't add any more creatine (a.k.a. water) to the system, and represents the end of the loading phase. If we continued to attempt to load, we'll not only waste our supplement and money, but possibly increase creatine clearance rate or reduce muscle transporter quantity (recall that creatine has to be transported into tissues, and any reduction in the number of transporters could subsequently hinder uptake).

In order to minimize any negative effects and maximize our cost efficiency, it is now our goal to use as little water as possible in an effort to keep the barrel full.

In the previous example we used a leak quantity of 1 cup per day. So in order to keep the barrel topped off, this would mean that we only have to add one cup a day to make up for this loss. Clearly this is a small and insignificant quantity.

Loaded: Reality

Using a quantity of 1 cup a day for leakage makes for nice math, but the reality is that this quantity might just be too high. Water leakage can occur at a slower rate, particularly on non-training days. This means that the amount of creatine used by our body on a daily basis is relatively small. That is evidenced by the fact that a creatine loaded individual can maintain elevated muscle creatine levels for more than a month after supplementation is discontinued!

In keeping with our minimalist theme, this all means that we only need to supplement with more creatine after we have caused a more significant depletion -such as after physical activity. Additionally, this could result in a training-induced elevation in creatine uptake, similar to the way in which glucose uptake is enhanced. Coupled with the insulin spike created by the post-workout meal, and the fact that creatine levels otherwise remain high, it is clear that the best time to use these supplements is post-exercise.

The Creatine Matrix Reloaded

Some people find that it is beneficial to reload on supplements every few months. If such a practice yields benefits, just as the initial loading phase did, it is indicative of sub-optimal doses being used in the maintenance phase. It is a good idea to try a reload after 6-8 weeks to test whether current maintenance doses are adequate.

Quick Tip: Fish oil may seem like a loading supplement, but for now it seems as though a consistent usage pattern is optimal.

Specifics

The above barrel example was merely used to illustrate how creatine loading works, and did not use any specific dosages. The cup of water example is not useable, so let's take a look at specific protocols for optimizing the loading supplements.

Creatine

Loading (if used): 10g (in 2 divided doses) for 2 weeks
Maintenance: 5g after physical activity
Reload (test): 10g (in 2 divided doses) for 1 week

Beta Alanine

Loading: 10g (in 2 divided doses) for 3 weeks
Maintenance: 6g (in 2 divided doses)
Reload (test): 10g (in 2 divided doses) for 4 days

*Creatine is used for examples because we have far more information about it than we do beta alanine.

Selected References

Derave W, Eijnde BO, Verbessem P, Ramaekers M, Van Leemputte M, Richter EA, Hespel P. Combined creatine and protein supplementation in conjunction with resistance training promotes muscle GLUT-4 content and glucose tolerance in humans. J Appl Physiol. 2003 May;94(5):1910-6.

Hultman E, Soderlund K, Timmons JA, Cederblad G, Greenhaff PL. Muscle creatine loading in men.J Appl Physiol. 1996 Jul;81(1):232-7.

Tarnopolsky M, Parise G, Fu MH, Brose A, Parshad A, Speer O, Wallimann T. Acute and moderate-term creatine monohydrate supplementation does not affect creatine transporter mRNA or protein content in either young or elderly humans. Mol Cell Biochem. 2003 Feb;244(1-2):159-66.

Vandenberghe K, Goris M, Van Hecke P, Van Leemputte M, Vangerven L, Hespel P. Long-term creatine intake is beneficial to muscle performance during resistance training. J Appl Physiol. 1997 Dec;83(6):2055-63.

Willott CA, Young ME, Leighton B, Kemp GJ, Boehm EA, Radda GK, Clarke K. Creatine uptake in isolated soleus muscle: kinetics and dependence on sodium, but not on insulin. Acta Physiol Scand. 1999 Jun;166(2):99-104.

Optimizing Post-Workout Nutrition

A variation on the review of whey protein, this section combines ideal timing with the optimal supplements to achieve the greatest possible anabolism.

What Are They?

Pre and post-workout nutrition are collectively referred to as para-workout nutrition. This involves special supplemented meals consumed at specific calculated times, and is one of the basics that initiated The Anabolic Index. Although post-workout nutrition is far more popular, it remains interesting that pre-workout nutrition is greatly superior in its effect. Even more powerful is the combination of the timing to yield the optimum anabolic effect.

Note: All drinks are based on the formula presented in "Designing The Ultimate Protein Drink".

Pre-Workout Power

Pre-workout meals are so powerful because they are quickly absorbed, and these nutrients are delivered to the working muscle during the exercise. This is critical because the elevated blood flow that occurs during training will enhance the amount of nutrient delivery, which in turn enhances anabolism. The best part is that the carbohydrate-containing pre-workout drink will stimulate insulin secretion, which elevates blood flow even more. This means that the synergistic effect between exercise and insulin-mediated blood flow will optimize muscle growth.

A (Not So) Hard Sell

It is often difficult for people to conceptualize that doing something before a workout can actually assist with during *and* post-workout anabolism, and this is likely why post-workout drinks have superior popularity. It is particularly interesting that in spite of the current hype surrounding blood flow stimulating supplements, which have never been shown to work at all, pre-workout meals are not considered a staple. What's more is that pre-workout drinks are the only supplementation shown to greatly increase blood flow and anabolism!

Post-Workout Power

The classic anabolic complement to training, post workout drinks help to restore muscle glycogen, and synergistically augment the anabolic training effect. By using carbohydrates post-workout, we stimulate the hormone insulin to act as the protein shield, as discussed in the section on Protein Protection. This helps to ensure that all of your high quality protein is utilized for the repair and synthesis of muscle. As an added bonus, the insulin also helps to stimulate amino acid entry into muscle, which further enhances the anabolic effect. Finally, although it is not necessary at this stage, the insulin assists carbohydrate entry into muscle, which facilitates glycogen replenishment.

It is important to understand that the body's carbohydrate tolerance is greatly enhanced following physical activity. This means that any carbohydrates provided by subsequent meals will be sucked up by muscle, rather than deposited as fat.

Quick Tip: Post-workout nutrition can be used by anyone, regardless if they use protein supplements or not. In fact, my most popular tip for sports teams is that they use chocolate milk after training and games (before the beer). It is readily available, tastes great, and provides the protein and carbohydrates to assist with recovery.

Double Post-Workout Power

The beauty with Protein Pulse Feeding is that a second post-workout drink may be consumed after the first, which will nearly double the anabolic effect! This is once again due to the synergy that exists between the amino acid Pulse and the post-training state. Addition of fast carbohydrates is not warranted at this time, which might reduce the anabolic impact (marginally), but avoids any potential bodyfat gain. There is plenty of time for growth so there is no need for excessive carbs here.

Practical Application: Acute Quantity

The quantity of sugars required for optimal anabolism and recovery is far lower than once thought, which allows us to maintain anabolism while avoiding any undesirable effects.

The actual amount of carbs consumed will be approximately 60g total divided between pre and post-workout for every hour of resistance training performed (for a 200lb individual). This number represents a moderately depleting workout, such as an intense chest and back session. The number will be smaller for lighter training (e.g. arms), and higher for intense leg or whole body sessions.

Any cardio or other anaerobic training will increase the necessary quantity by 50% per hour –again, this is intensity dependent. For example, an added hour of cardio would necessitate an additional 30g of carbohydrates, brining the total to 90g.

For multiple post workout Protein Pulse Feedings, only the first meal will contain any significant amount of carbs. Subsequent liquid meals should use less than 15g of carbohydrate for Protein Protection, while limiting the insulin response. Due to the amount of insulin stimulated before and shortly after training, it is undesirable to stimulate this hormone any further. Finally, the carbohydrate in subsequent liquid meals can be sucrose (as opposed to glucose or maltodextrin), which will ensure that the drink tastes better and is less likely to induce a large insulin release.

Practical Application: Timing

Another important factor we need to consider is nutrient timing. In order to maximize anabolism and recovery, the meals should be consumed such that both physical and nutrient performance is optimized.

Pre-workout meals should be consumed within 10-15 minutes of training. If the meal is consumed earlier then insulin may spike and a decrease in blood sugar could occur. If the drink is consumed later, then it may cause an undesirable fullness during training.

Post-workout meals should be consumed 10-15 minutes after training. This is because of the temporary state of protein resistance, known as the Post-Workout Blackout period, that occurs immediately after training. Essentially, this is a time when the amino acid induction of protein synthesis (a.k.a. Protein Potential) is hindered. It is unknown why this protein resistance occurs immediately after a workout, but waiting for a short time after is warranted. This is covered in more detail in Anabolic Myth #3.

Secondary post-workout meals are consumed 0.75-1 hour after the first, if whey hydrolysate is used. This timing is largely dictated by the blood sugar response of the first post-workout drink. Ideally, one would sip on sugar water for 10-20 minutes, starting 30 minutes after the first drink. Then, 1-1.25 hours after the first drink, the second would be consumed. Again, this is ideal, but impractical for all but the strictest of athletes.

Timing Summary

10-15min pre-drink ⇒ Training ⇒ 10-15 minutes post #1 ⇒ 45-60min later post #2

Protein Intake

Due to the critical importance of this factor it has been discussed in detail under the sections "Whey Protein" and "Designing The Ultimate Protein Drink".

Quick Tip: A lot of people ask about pre-made sports drinks for consumption during and after a workout. Although they do provide a small quantity of electrolytes, this is easily accomplished by adding a little table salt (which helps with creatine uptake anyway) to your own drink. Additionally, the carbohydrate source is inferior compared to one that we could make using a sugar free flavored beverage and our own ingredients (such as glucose or maltodextrin). Finally, studies have shown that such drinks will only help performance if it persists for 90 minutes or more, which is beyond the duration of most activity.

Selected References

Borsheim E, Tipton KD, Wolf SE, Wolfe RR. Essential amino acids and muscle protein recovery from resistance exercise. Am J Physiol Endocrinol Metab. 2002 Oct;283(4):E648-57.

Calbet JA, MacLean DA. Plasma glucagon and insulin responses depend on the rate of appearance of amino acids after ingestion of different protein solutions in humans. J Nutr. 2002 Aug;132(8):2174-82.

Koopman R, Beelen M, Stellingwerff T, Pennings B, Saris WH, Kies AK, Kuipers H, van Loon LJ. Coingestion of carbohydrate with protein does not further augment postexercise muscle protein synthesis. Am J Physiol Endocrinol Metab. **2007 Sep;293(3):E833-42**

Rasmussen, BB, Tipton KD, Miller SL, Wolf SE, and Wolfe RR. An oral essential amino acid-carbohydrate supplement enhances muscle protein anabolism after resistance exercise. J Appl Physiol 88: 386-392, 2000

Tipton KD, Rasmussen BB, Miller SL, Wolf SE, Owens-Stovall SK, Petrini BE, Wolfe RR. Timing of amino acid-carbohydrate ingestion alters anabolic response of muscle to resistance exercise. Am J Physiol Endocrinol Metab. 2001 Aug;281(2):E197-206

Tipton KD, Borsheim E, Wolf SE, Sanford AP, Wolfe RR Acute response of net muscle protein balance reflects 24-h balance after exercise and amino acid ingestion. Am J Physiol Endocrinol Metab. 2003 Jan;284(1):E76-89.

van Loon LJ, Saris WH, Verhagen H, Wagenmakers AJ. Plasma insulin responses after ingestion of different amino acid or protein mixtures with carbohydrate. Am J Clin Nutr. 2000 Jul;72(1):96-105.

For Advanced Athletes Only

Optimization is the key to The Anabolic Index, and this has never been truer than it is with regard to para-workout nutrition. To make things even better we've had a couple of relatively recent developments in this area that will make a tremendous difference in our performance and muscle growth. But I must warn that these substances are for advanced athletes only, due to the rigor with which their care must be maintained.

Rather than sounding like ad copy, these supplements aren't "too powerful", or any such nonsense. Rather they are expensive and should be considered very high maintenance.

NOTE: Due to the limited number of people who benefit greatly from these supplements, only a brief overview is made here.

Getting Faster

The benefit of these supplements is that they are absorbed faster than anything else we have on the market today. This means that we'll have greater precision when Protein Pulse Feeding, or during para-workout nutrition.

The Protein

The first such ingredient is a type of whey protein that is fractionated into such small parts that it is essentially di- and tri-peptides, which means strings of two or three amino acids bound together. This is optimal because our body specifically absorbs these small peptides and does not have to break them down any farther.

Additionally, this means freeing up amino acid transporters so in all, we're getting quicker absorption than would otherwise occur. So far I am only aware of one company that makes this product and they are based out of Europe (although it is also sold in North America).

The Carbohydrate

Waxy maize starch is an interesting carbohydrate because it has a large molecular structure, yet has been shown to be absorbed more quickly than our other gold standard sugars (i.e. glucose and maltodextrin). More importantly, this carbohydrate has been shown to induce an optimal rate of glycogen storage – again, beyond anything else we have.

The Downside

As previously mentioned, there products are expensive and great care must be taken with their use. This is because their rates of absorption are so high that they can induce a blood sugar or protein crash, such that our blood glucose and amino acid levels drop below what is optimal. This is greatly catabolic, not to mention unhealthy, and must be avoided at all costs.

Timing

Using the template from the previous section we can apply the new products and come up with a slightly different timing scheme. Specifically, post-workout drinks should be separated by no more than 30 minutes in order to avoid a blood sugar crash. It is critical that one be vigilant about monitoring blood sugar until a personal understanding of how such a drink affects that individual is developed.

Due to the rapid nature of these ingredients, their use in pre-workout nutrition is not warranted for training that lasts 45 minutes or longer. Otherwise, the standard guidelines apply.

Quick Tip: In terms of human performance and function, these ingredients are a great alternative to pre-made sports drinks, although the ability to mix in water and taste are not ideal.

Case Study: A Users Guide to Pre-Workout Meals

Brian had read about the benefits of pre-workout meals for months and finally decided to give them a try. At 6'0 and a lean 250lbs, Brian wasn't exactly new to the lifting game, but this experience almost put him back to square one.

He started out with his usual pre-workout ritual steel cut oats and tuna, eaten an hour before training. Just before the workout, he consumed 60g of whey protein and 70g of sucrose (table sugar). Then it was off to train legs.

It was after only the second set of squats that Brian knew he was in trouble. All of that food sitting on his stomach during the most demanding exercise of the week had caught up to him... very quickly.

That same day he contacted me about this horrible experience, saying that he was never going to try pre-workout meals again. Although I tried to be positive, Brian had made numerous errors that needed to be corrected. Here are the problems we discussed with his pre-workout meal:

1) Having a solid meal so close to his workout

Eating solid food just 60 minutes before training is cutting it close for most people. In fact, if you're consuming solid food, you're much better off eating it 2 hours pre-training. That way you'll benefit from the nutrients during your workout, but you won't have the sluggish feeling of food sitting in your gut while trying to sit and then stand up with 500lbs on your back.

2) Having a pre-workout drink despite a recent solid meal

The idea behind pre-workout nutrition is that it supplies our muscle with amino acids during a time of increased blood flow to that tissue. Although a liquid pre-workout meal is far more precise, and certainly more anabolic due to insulin, you don't need a drink if you've eaten within 2 hours of your workout.

A solid meal consumed a couple of hours before training would have prevented a situation of muscle breakdown during the workout, and may have even caused a little muscle growth -albeit far less than a liquid meal. The Anabolic Index is about optimization so liquid meals are always recommended, *but* it is also about optimization for YOU and YOUR lifestyle. So if it's not feasible to time your meals perfectly throughout the day, so that you have a pre-workout liquid meal, then a solid meal at the appropriate time is reasonable alternative.

3) Using whey concentrate

Early on in the history of whey proteins it was believed that whey in general was considered "fast". What this means is that it gets into our gut and is ready for use relatively soon after it is consumed. While this "fast" designation may stand against conventional proteins, we now have a new benchmark for speed: amino acids. Because they do not have to be digested, amino acids are simply absorbed and are available for use quite quickly. This means that whey protein in general is really an <u>intermediate speed</u> for our purposes, because there is digestion time to be considered.

The exception to this rule is whey hydrolysate, which is also fast because it is whey protein that has been chemically pre-digested. In addition to single amino acids, our body can absorb very small groups of protein (called di- and tri-peptides), of which whey hydrolysate is largely comprised.

4) Using sucrose

Much like protein, we don't want to use a carbohydrate source that has to be digested. Although sucrose is considered a simple sugar, it still has to be digested and even metabolized before it can be fully used. If you've been following the theme of speed, you'll quickly realize that sucrose is not the ideal carbohydrate for our pre-workout purposes. Instead, glucose (also known as dextrose or sometimes even "corn sugar") is what we want to use because it is simply absorbed without having to be broken down or converted to anything else. The sugar called maltodextrin will also work optimally, although it is slightly more difficult to acquire.

5) First attempt on leg day

Even with an iron stomach, I'd never suggest that anyone try a pre-workout drink for the first time on leg day. It is usually on this training day that we recruit the greatest amount of muscle mass by performing deadlifts, squats, and cleans. In other words, the stresses on our body are greatest on this day. This means that we will be more likely to have a negative reaction with something on our stomach —even if it's only water.

6) Full drink first time

As another precautionary measure for those who may be especially sensitive, it is best to start with smaller doses of pre-workout drinks and then work your way up to a full 1L of liquid.

Considerations For The Ultimate Protein Drink

If we're trying to make a protein shake that's going to optimize our muscle growth and recovery, there are numerous factors that need to be taken into consideration -the most important of which is the purpose of the drink. Once you figure out exactly what you want the drink to do, then you can go ahead and figure out how to do it. Don't worry, all of the guesswork has been taken out and by the end of it all, you're left with the basic formulae.

Goals? To Build Muscle!

Naturally the main goal is going to be the same, but we have to consider the timing of the drink in question. Namely, is this a drink that is going to be consumed before a workout, or it is something we're consuming before we sleep. The implications of such a question are enormous, because they yield precisely opposite formulations.

The Difference is Night and Day

So what makes day and night drinks so completely different? Fundamentally, it is the speed at which they are absorbed in our gut. This is critical because we want day drinks to be absorbed quickly, and night drinks absorbed slowly. The former is critical in order to generate a Protein Pulse and stimulate anabolism (Anabolic Index **Key #2**). Night drinks on the other hand, are designed to slow digestion because they have to supply nutrients throughout the highly catabolic overnight fast (Anabolic Index **Key #3**).

Initial Considerations

So how do we design such different drinks? It's not all that complicated once you know what to look for.

1) Dilution

Often overlooked when designing drinks, dilution is of critical importance for speed of absorption. Dilute solutions will be absorbed more quickly than thicker drinks.

2) Volume

Related to dilution, we need to adjust the volume of liquid according to both the quantity of nutrients and desired effect. Additionally, volume is of consideration pre-exercise and pre-sleep.

3) Protein Choice

Perhaps the most important factor, speed of protein is critical to the purpose of the drink. A rapidly absorbed drink, that does not require digestion, is ideal for precision manipulation of muscle growth. Conversely, a slower digesting protein shake is optimal for what would otherwise be a prolonged fast.

4) Fat and Carbohydrate Content

Protein shakes are rarely consumed without the addition of different nutrient-containing ingredients. This could be something as simple as fruit or peanut butter, but the effects are dramatically different.

5) Timing

As the most obvious factor for consideration, the time at which the drink is consumed should be well thought out.

6) Other Supplements (creatine, beta-alanine)

Often the consumption of other supplements accompanies that of a protein drink. For this to be worthwhile they should complement each other without any hindrance on any of the above factors.

Summary of Factors

	Day Drink	**Night Drink**
Dilution	Dilute	Thick
Volume	High	Low
Protein	Fast	Slow
Nutrients	Carbs	Fats
Timing	Pre/Post-Workout	Before Sleep
Additions	Creatine, Beta-alanine, BCAA	Fish Oil, BCAA

Designing The Ultimate Protein Drink

The Day Shake*

1.2 Liter water

40g Whey Hydrolysate

25g Glucose (a.k.a. Dextrose a.k.a. Corn Sugar) or Maltodextrin

10g BCAA

5g Creatine monohydrate

5g Beta alanine

Rationale

The high volume is necessary to ensure optimal dilution for quick absorption, which affords a degree of nutrient timing precision. Whey hydrolysate is used because it is the most rapidly absorbed protein, due to the fact that it does not have to be greatly digested. Naturally, this rapid absorption induces a Protein Pulse and subsequently muscle growth.

Similarly, the carbohydrate source is rapidly absorbed to ensure an insulin spike, which is important for glycogen restoration in the morning and post-workout, or the pre-workout stimulation of blood flow. Most importantly, the insulin minimizes the amount of protein wasted by oxidation (Protein Protection), resulting in improved protein utilization.

BCAA use will facilitate protein synthesis, and make use of the protective effect of insulin. Creatine uptake is best after exercise when natural stores are depleted, when the insulin will force more into muscle. Beta alanine is best used after a workout when stores are depleted and may make use of the protective effect of carbohydrate-induced insulin.

No fats are used in the time surrounding the workout because they slow digestion, and will greatly disrupt what we are trying to achieve.

Day Shake: Special Considerations

As mentioned in the review of whey hydrolysate, this protein generally tastes horrible. This is of concern when multiple drinks per day are warranted, and even getting it down can be a challenge for some. The sugars will help, but making foul items sweet isn't always a great idea (as I found out when I once added sucrose to the liver on my plate). If the flavor becomes an issue, then using only a pre-workout and possibly waking drink is warranted. Whey isolate can be used post workout if necessary, and although this is not ideal, <u>it is more important to follow some of the optimal protocol than simply reject the entire plan due to rigidity</u>.

It is also important to note that the sugars will spike blood sugar and insulin (a good thing for growth and recovery), which could ultimately result in a blood sugar crash if carbohydrates (from the next meal) are not consumed within an appropriate time. This is easily avoidable and should always be prevented.

The Night Shake*

500mL water

80g Casein

20g Olive or Flax Oil

10g BCAA

3g Fish Oil

*Quantities based on a 200lb individual.

Rationale

The low volume and dilution will ensure that the nutrients are slowly distributed to the body during sleep. Also, it is important that the volume be kept small to minimize stomach discomfort when lying down. Casein is a slow-digesting protein that will, along with dilution, feed the body throughout the otherwise fasted time.

The quantity of casein is higher than those that are commonly recommended, which erroneously use the amount of protein desired in a typical meal. This does not account for the fact that this single meal is meant to feed the body for 8 hours. Such recommendations are particularly surprising when you consider that many people believe sleep to be such an anabolic time (see Myths Section for more information). In reality, sleep is not very anabolic, but we still need to feed the body during this time.

In contrast to the day shake, fats replace carbohydrates in the night drink. The reasons for this are two fold: 1) The way in which our body responds to carbohydrates is generally compromised at night, and 2) Fat will be the final piece of the puzzle to ensure that digestion does not happen any faster than desired. Much like carbohydrates, the added fat will serve to protect the protein from unnecessary breakdown before it is used.

BCAA's are used for their anticatabolic properties at night, because they are often required for energy production during this time, which means that the body would tear apart entire proteins in order to get at them. If they are supplied by night supplementation this will spare muscle from being broken down.

Other Considerations

The above examples highlight some of the things you can do to optimize your nutrition, but there are always numerous variables that only you can account for. Using pre workout drinks as an example, the volume would have to be adjusted, taking into consideration the type of workout that is going to be performed -often 1.2 L of water is just too much, even if all the necessary precautions are taken (see "The Protein FAQ" section for more information).

Quick Tip: For a wide variety of protein shakes, be sure to check out the final section of this manual!

FAQ. Your [sic] wrong. I know I need more carbs post-workout.

A. As mentioned in the Other Considerations section (above), these are only examples and not meant to be replicated or used in every situation. Carbohydrate content will vary depending on factors such as: the rest of your daily carbohydrate intake, whether you had a pre-workout drink, and the type and intensity of exercise performed.

Clearly someone who performs hard physical activity (e.g. playing a sport) for an hour will need more carbohydrates than someone who performs a biceps workout. In fact, resistance training does not deplete glycogen stores very much compared to other forms of activity, which should be a consideration for pre and post-workout nutrition. Most importantly, no single drink example can satisfy every possible situation.

SEVEN

The Protein FAQ II

"Sometimes it takes a crazy person to see the truth. If so, I'm a freaking lunatic."
-Stephen Colbert

3. How Much Protein Can We Digest At One Time?

You may have heard the old rumor that you can only digest 30 grams of protein in one sitting. In fact, this old wives tale is so prominent that I've spouted it off numerous times myself (back when I was a training novice). Of course the 30-gram quantity is completely arbitrary, but it really does raise the question of how much protein we can digest at one sitting. But is this asking the right question? Is the act of digestion really limiting to our efficient use of ingested protein?

We know that humans can't ingest an unlimited amount of protein without having some kind of regulation. In our attempt to find the solution, consider the following:

Digestion→ Absorption→ Metabolism→ Excretion

This figure shows the path through which our nutrients travel, once ingested. Much like links in the chain, we should consider each segment to figure out where the limit lies.

i) **Digestion**: The 30-gram myth is silly, and we don't have any reason to suspect that digestion is a limiting factor in healthy people.

ii) **Absorption**: If the amount of protein that our gut can absorb were limiting, then we would simply have the excess protein stuck in the digestion stage waiting to be digested. This would mean that we could consume 200 grams of protein in one sitting and simply have it feed our body for the remainder of the day. Clearly this doesn't happen, so although absorption may be limiting at an extreme, there is a more important part of the story than this.

iii) **Metabolism**: If our ability to metabolize (biochemically "handle") protein and amino acids were limiting, then it would mean that excessive protein is digested and absorbed, but our body would deal with it in such a way that it is not used. In fact, this is exactly what happens. You may know of this process by another name: oxidation. Fortunately, **Key #5** of The Anabolic Index (Protein Protection) shows us how to ensure that even when we consume high amounts of protein, our body makes use of it as efficiently as possible: for muscle growth.

We may not know exactly how much protein can be metabolized at once (this depends on too many factors including, protein speed, hormonal and training states, as well as Caloric intake), it is a safe bet that we will be burning off some protein most of the time. Considering that **Key #4** suggests that we consume an excess amount of protein for optimal body composition. Quantifying protein digestion is irrelevant for most people.

Quick Tip: As a general guideline, remember that the faster the protein source, the more likely it is to be oxidized if consumed in excess.

Selected References

Arnal MA, Mosoni L, Boirie Y, Houlier ML, Morin L, Verdier E, Ritz P, Antoine JM, Prugnaud J, Beaufrere B, Mirand PP. Protein pulse feeding improves protein retention in elderly women. Am J Clin Nutr. 1999 Jun;69(6):1202-8

Elia M, Khan K, Jennings G. Effect of mixed meal ingestion on fuel utilization in the whole body and in superficial and deep forearm tissues. Br J Nutr. 1999 May;81(5):373-81

Koopman R, Wagenmakers AJ, Manders RJ, Zorenc AH, Senden JM, Gorselink M, Keizer HA, van Loon LJ. Combined ingestion of protein and free leucine with carbohydrate increases postexercise muscle protein synthesis in vivo in male subjects. Am J Physiol Endocrinol Metab. 2005 Apr;288(4):E645-53

Pacy PJ, Price GM, Halliday D, Quevedo MR, Millward DJ. Nitrogen homeostasis in man: the diurnal responses of protein synthesis and degradation and amino acid oxidation to diets with increasing protein intakes. Clin Sci (Lond). 1994 Jan;86(1):103-16.

Rasmussen BB, Tipton KD, Miller SL, Wolf SE, Wolfe RR. An oral essential amino acid-carbohydrate supplement enhances muscle protein anabolism after resistance exercise. J Appl Physiol. 2000 Feb;88(2):386-92

Tipton KD, Ferrando AA, Phillips SM, Doyle D Jr, Wolfe RR. Postexercise net protein synthesis in human muscle from orally administered amino acids. Am J Physiol. 1999 Apr;276(4 Pt 1):E628-34

4. Is It Good To Drink My Protein During A Workout?

This was a common practice several years ago that seemed like a good idea at the time. More recently it has been discovered that this practice is actually suboptimal, and there are several reasons why this is so:

i) Gut Bloodflow

The most obvious reason hindering consumption of nutrients during a workout is that blood flow to the gut is greatly reduced during exercise. This makes sense because we know that at this time our body is focused on performance, rather than digesting something. With reduced digestion and absorption activity, we're less likely to get the nutrients we need, <u>and</u> cause unnecessary gastric discomfort.

Contrary to consuming the liquid meal pre-workout, which can be largely absorbed before exercise gets intense, workout meals consumed during training will not be absorbed as well.

ii) The Accommodation Response

Let's go back to **Key #2** of The Anabolic Index, which is Protein Pulse Feeding. This is used to not only to stimulate protein synthesis, but also to avoid the accommodation response (i.e. a state of protein resistance induced by prolonged amino acid exposure), which may occur when sipping a protein beverage. By sipping a protein drink throughout our workout, we're providing a steady stream of amino acids into our bloodstream, which results in this negative accommodation response.

Quick Tip: It is the pulsing of protein, much like the pulsing of a heartbeat, which helps to maximally stimulate muscle growth. An amino acid flatline, just like a flatline heartbeat, signals the death of protein synthesis.

iii) The Post-Workout Blackout Period

The Post-Workout Blackout Period is a time of protein resistance that occurs immediately after training. This is why waiting for a short period of time before consumption is warranted. Unfortunately, when we sip our protein drink during training, much of the absorption occurs during this questionable time (immediately after exercise), not during the exercise session itself! Remember that it takes time for the drink to go from our mouth to our bloodstream, especially during vigorous physical activity.

What's worse is that we don't know when this blackout period begins, so if it begins during our workout (which in all likelihood it does), we're providing our body with amino acids during a time that we are insensitive to their powerful effects.

iv) The Insulin Response

Much of the power of pre-workout nutrition lies in the ability to stimulate insulin before training. The resulting effect is known as "Priming the Pump", which is enhancement of the bloodflow and subsequent nutrient delivery to muscle. This means that more nutrients are reaching our working tissue, and increasing protein synthesis to a greater degree.

Now this effect happens most effectively when the pre-workout drink consists of both protein and carbohydrates. By consuming the entire drink within a short period of time we maximize the protein pulsing and insulin stimulating effects. Unfortunately, when sipping a beverage (which some people suggest during a workout), the insulin response is blunted, thus minimizing the blood flow and anabolic effects.

Quick Tip: Consumption during a workout may be beneficial if the drink is sufficiently dilute and the activity persists for more that 90 minutes. In this case a commercial sports drink may be an acceptable option, although a homemade version is less expensive and more efficacious.

5. Is It Okay To Premix Protein Shakes?

For the sake of convenience, many people like to make up all of their protein shakes for the day at one time. That way, when it's time for a drink, it's ready to go.

As great of a timesaver as this may be the question remains about the stability of protein in water (or whatever beverage you use). Does the protein break down from sitting in water for too long? Likely not. In fact it takes a very powerful acid to unravel a typical tightly wound protein, and only then do specific enzymes have the ability to break it down during natural digestion.

Our drinks contain neither powerful acid (we hope) or enzymes, the drinks are likely safe from breakdown for several hours (preferably refrigerated). Now even if the drinks were simply broken down, they could be broken into amino acids to enhance the speed of absorption. This would actually be a good thing, unless we're talking about the slow digesting evening or nocturnal shakes. Realistically speaking however, protein breakdown into its component amino acids is unlikely.

The real reason you wouldn't want to go for more than 12 hours is that the protein may be susceptible to damage from oxygen, which may convert the amino acids into a less useable form. There also exists the possibility of microbial growth in the drink, which is why I wouldn't use protein that has been in liquid form for more than 5 hours unrefrigerated. This amount of time is largely based on my experience with milk products (and subsequent time in the microbiology lab), but better safe than sorry. Having said that, it's best to use your own judgment on this one.

Quick Tip: Remember that the anabolic potential of these drinks can also apply to microorganisms. Having opened a protein shake container that has been sitting in my basement for a couple of weeks, I can personally attest to this. Keep your stored protein drinks refrigerated if possible, and always in an airtight container. This should limit both the amount of oxidation and potential microbial growth.

EIGHT

7 Anabolic Myths

"It's not so much what you have to learn if you accept weird theories, it's what you have to unlearn."
-Isaac Asimov

Myth 1. Insulin is the Most Anabolic Hormone

This is a <u>paradoxical myth</u>, a true statement that has been bastardized to the point that the meaning is incorrect or skewed. In other words, although the actual statement may be true in some sense, for our practical purposes it is false. Using our insulin example, it is in fact the most anabolic hormone in our body, but not in the way that most of us think.

What Does "Anabolic" Mean?

The term anabolic simply refers to an energy consuming process that builds a bigger molecule out of smaller molecules. The most commonly imagined example of an anabolic process is the building of muscle tissue out of protein/amino acids. We know that this type of anabolism both uses energy (and lots of it) and combines smaller amino acids into larger proteins.

The problem is that insulin is the most anabolic hormone, not because it builds muscle tissue the best, but because it is anabolic to *all* of the macronutrients, not just protein. Stated another way, insulin is great at storing fat and carbohydrates in our body.

Just take a look at an individual with chronically elevated testosterone compared to someone with elevated insulin levels. The difference in their physiques alone will verify how "anabolic" each hormone can be.

Of course insulin can be made use of for enhanced glycogen storage and muscle protein synthesis, by timing of specific spikes (e.g. post-workout), but chronically elevated levels of this hormone are highly undesirable (for health as well as body composition purposes).

To sum up; insulin is anabolic by storing *all* macronutrients, including fats and carbohydrates -it is this unique property, NOT enhanced muscle building activity, that makes it the most anabolic hormone.

Quick Tip: In the morning and after a workout, insulin will be more anabolic to muscle and less anabolic to fat cells. This is one reason why we take advantage of these times in The Anabolic Index.

Case Study: Insulin As The Most Anabolic Hormone

Nathan was a screwed up teenager who wanted to do everything in his power to get big —everything except eat properly. He read that insulin was the most anabolic hormone in his body, and since it was both legal and easy to access, he thought he'd give it a try. Horrible (over)training and worse eating led to a gradual accumulation of bodyfat, and over the course of nearly 2 years, a nice layer was covering his body.

In spite of eventually cleaning up his act, including his authorship of a widely circulated article series on how to best use insulin while minimizing bodyfat (which is still quite popular today), the once ripped physique grew to "unfortunate" proportions —nearly all of it body fat, the rest being insulin-enhanced glycogen storage, NOT actual muscle.

Of course he had blood sugar crashes, and the potential damage to his health remains to this day, but overall it changed forever the way he would view the most anabolic hormone.

Myth 2. Sleep Is The Most Anabolic Time for Recovery

Perhaps the oldest and most pervasive myth still in existence, the concept of sleep as our main anabolic time has been defying reason for decades. This idea stems from several factors; the most noteworthy (and simple) is that we feel like garbage if we don't get enough sleep. Also when we're sleep deprived: performance declines, cortisol levels increase, and testosterone falls though the floor. That's a pretty bad situation to be in.

What About Growth Hormone?

One of the biggest arguments for the anabolic potential of sleep has to do with growth hormone (GH) release. We know that the levels of this very anabolic hormone are highest when we sleep. So clearly GH makes sleep anabolic, right?

Unfortunately not, because the catabolic hormone cortisol is secreted in concert with GH, and largely negates any anabolic effect. In fact, this relationship may be predominantly catabolic depending on the circumstances.

But What About Soreness?

Some also argue that we don't feel sore after a workout unless we get enough sleep, and since soreness means that we're growing, sleep is anabolic. Well soreness itself isn't necessarily anabolic, but that's a whole can of worms to open another time. The most important thing to take away from this idea is that at best, a lack of sleep is negative for growth –*there is still no suggestion that sleep itself is positively <u>anabolic</u>*.

The difference is that sleep is a natural phenomenon that normally occurs, and it is the *absence* of this process that is negative. Its presence just means that things are running normally, not that this process itself is positive; merely neutral. It's like having a car without gas –it could be called "slow" (to put it mildly). Now does this mean that adding gas makes the car "fast", or does adding gas just bring it up to normal?

The Nightmare of Catabolism

Okay, so getting enough sleep allows for the prevention of some anti-anabolic symptoms, but does that mean that sleep itself is actually anabolic? Now I'm not suggesting for a minute that sleep isn't important. It certainly is, but there's another angle from which to look at the picture; sleep is largely catabolic. That's right, rather than being anabolic, sleep is actually the time of our greatest muscle breakdown.

Going back to our construction analogy, we know that we need three things for muscle growth and repair:

1) Building Materials
2) Signal to Build
3) Energy (this is a new one, but it's just intuitive)

So how much of each do we have when we sleep? We may have the signal to build muscle if we've trained recently, but how about the other two. Well, even if you're consuming a slow protein before bed, you may run out of building materials (amino acids) before you wake. If not, then it's at least clear that we won't have optimal amino acid levels for anabolism. This also applies for energy because we're ultimately fasted before morning. So even if we only needed two out of three requirements for muscle growth, we *still* wouldn't be in an anabolic phase.

So how does this make sleep catabolic? Unfortunately for us, muscle breakdown isn't as picky -it only needs *one* signal. What's worse is that the absence of the other two necessary anabolic components (building materials and energy) automatically starts the signal for breakdown. In other words, if we don't have enough energy or protein in our body, we'll enter a catabolic situation for muscle. Of course this happens to nearly all of us every single night.

Training and Protein Intake

What's worse is that training itself, while a stimulus for muscle growth, is also a stimulus for muscle catabolism. This paradoxical effect can be explained by the fact that our body has to breakdown old and worn out tissue caused by training. Now if we're well-fed, then this isn't a problem. But if we're fasted, it's a horrible situation.

As a final kick in the teeth, our body doesn't just break down muscle so that our vital organs like our heart and brain can function. Our body actually breaks down our muscle to supply other tissues with amino acids –most notably our gut. And don't forget that our high, albeit optimal, protein intake may exacerbate the whole process!

So despite all of the horrible effects of sleep depravation, and despite the growth hormone pulses, it is clear that sleep is horribly catabolic. Fortunately part of The Anabolic Index deals with how to mitigate or even reverse these negative effects, as discussed in **Key #3** (Protein Withdrawal) and Designing The Ultimate Protein Shake.

Quick Tip: Optimal sleep can be achieved by practicing relaxation techniques and maintaining a consistent routine before bed. This will ensure a reduced state of arousal that is ideal for sleep.

Myth 3. There is a One Hour Post-Workout Window

Post-workout nutrition is a hot topic and has been for a number of years. The idea is that for a short time following resistance exercise, our body is more receptive to nutrients in order to facilitate recovery. This means that more ingested protein is stored as muscle, and more carbohydrates are stored as glycogen.

How Many Windows Are There?

The down side of the dogma is that most claim that a specific duration, or window of opportunity, exists for this enhanced period of recovery. Sadly, the concept has been so perverted such that in just one week of reading, I had read several different articles about the topic, all claiming a different duration of "window".

By far the most common duration, which has almost become a punch line for obsolescence, is the one-hour post-workout window. This is hyped up based on studies showing that post workout protein drinks have an enhanced effect on recovery if they are consumed immediately after exercise as opposed to if they were consumed some time later.

These studies had a huge impact on the way we looked at post-workout nutrition, and although their application is flawed, the impact has largely been positive. The fundamental flaw in the application of these studies is that they erroneously use study groups that do not necessarily apply to us (in this case).

Erroneous Application

Specifically, the most often cited study used elderly subjects and resistance training. It is important to understand that this group benefits from consuming their entire daily intake of protein in one single sitting -clearly disadvantageous to anyone using this manual.

The other research used to support the one-hour post-workout window idea, used cardiovascular exercise. Although this type of exercise increases muscle protein synthesis the ultimate outcome is clearly far different from someone who is resistance training.

In terms of knowledge acquisition, these studies should be followed when they are the only evidence available. So in order to consider them invalid, more directly applicable studies need to have been performed. Fortunately, they come from the lab in which I used to study, which is the same lab that provided the majority of evidence for optimizing muscle growth.

When examining studies performed on healthy people, it becomes clear that there is no real definable post-workout window. In fact, the more directly applicable research suggests that the enhanced responsiveness to post-workout nutrition lasts for more than 24 hours!

HINT: That's not a "window" at all!

Protein Resistance: The Post-Workout Blackout

With regard to the previously held notion that protein drinks consumed immediately after training provide the greatest benefit, it turns out that this is not only false, but likely counterproductive. In fact, applicable studies using healthy adults and resistance exercise show that there is a 30% smaller increase in protein synthesis when the drink is consumed immediately after, as opposed to one hour post training. This is tantamount to consuming the drink without the protein protection or other benefits of carbohydrates.

Reasons for this period of protein resistance, known as the post-workout blackout, are unknown, but may have to do with blood flow to the digestive tract during, and immediately following, training. Does that mean that we need to wait an hour to consume our post workout shake? Not at all. That was simply a time point used in a study rather than a suggestion for timing.

What About Carbs?

Another suggestion for drinking right after training is due to a potential enhanced glycogen replenishment during this time. This idea has little potential significance for athletes and those trying to build muscle, because glycogen restoration is easily enhanced simply as a consequence of optimizing muscle growth. In other words, if we just focus on optimizing the muscle building aspect of post-workout nutrition, then the glycogen restoration will just come along for the ride.

As an additional positive note, it turns out that muscle insulin sensitivity, which is a determining factor in the fate of ingested carbohydrates and protein, is enhanced for more than 24 hours following resistance exercise. This means that our body is more likely to use carbohydrates than it is to store them as fat.

Esoteric Science Note: Post-workout non-insulin-mediated glucose uptake cannot be used without the ingestion of rapidly absorbed carbohydrates, which ironically (in this case) stimulates insulin release.

The Updated Thinking

Considering that all of the adaptations that were once thought to be short lived have turned out to last for 24 hours or more, the idea of limiting a post-workout window is not longer valid. It's okay though, because the reality is even better than the myth.

It is better to think of the prolonged post-workout period as one of enhanced protein and insulin sensitivity, during which we can optimize recovery and body composition. With this line of thinking, we are better able to understand our own biochemistry and ensure that we're taking advantage of proper nutrition for ideal results.

Quick Tip: Although we don't know how long the post-workout blackout lasts, it is likely a manifestation of the stressed metabolic or digestive response during training. This means that waiting 15-20 minutes after training should get us out of the blackout period and into one of enhanced protein sensitivity.

FAQ. Your [sic] wrong. I drink my protein shake immediately after training and I know it helps.

A. The evidence doesn't suggest that drinking "as soon as the last weight hits the floor" is detrimental or will actually inhibit growth -in fact it's not a horrible idea, it's just sub optimal.

Selected References

Borsheim E, Tipton KD, Wolf SE, Wolfe RR. Essential amino acids and muscle protein recovery from resistance exercise. Am J Physiol Endocrinol Metab. 2002 Oct;283(4):E648-57.

Calbet JA, MacLean DA. Plasma glucagon and insulin responses depend on the rate of appearance of amino acids after ingestion of different protein solutions in humans. J Nutr. 2002 Aug;132(8):2174-82.

Esmarck B, Andersen JL, Olsen S, Richter EA, Mizuno M, Kjaer M. Timing of postexercise protein intake is important for muscle hypertrophy with resistance training in elderly humans. J Physiol. 2001 Aug 15;535(Pt 1):301-11.

Koopman R, Manders RJ, Zorenc AH, Hul GB, Kuipers H, Keizer HA, van Loon LJ. A single session of resistance exercise enhances insulin sensitivity for at least 24 h in healthy men. Eur J Appl Physiol. 2005 May;94(1-2):180-7.

Koopman R, Wagenmakers AJ, Manders RJ, Zorenc AH, Senden JM, Gorselink M, Keizer HA, van Loon LJ. Combined ingestion of protein and free leucine with carbohydrate increases postexercise muscle protein synthesis in vivo in male subjects. Am J Physiol Endocrinol Metab. 2005 Apr;288(4):E645-53.

Koopman R, Beelen M, Stellingwerff T, Pennings B, Saris WH, Kies AK, Kuipers H, van Loon LJ. Coingestion of carbohydrate with protein does not further augment postexercise muscle protein synthesis. Am J Physiol Endocrinol Metab. 2007 Sep;293(3):E833-42

Levenhagen DK, Gresham JD, Carlson MG, Maron DJ, Borel MJ, Flakoll PJ. Postexercise nutrient intake timing in humans is critical to recovery of leg glucose and protein homeostasis. Am J Physiol Endocrinol Metab. 2001 Jun;280(6):E982-93.

Rasmussen, BB, Tipton KD, Miller SL, Wolf SE, and Wolfe RR. An oral essential amino acid-carbohydrate supplement enhances muscle protein anabolism after resistance exercise. J Appl Physiol 88: 386-392, 2000

Tipton KD, Rasmussen BB, Miller SL, Wolf SE, Owens-Stovall SK, Petrini BE, Wolfe RR. Timing of amino acid-carbohydrate ingestion alters anabolic response of muscle to resistance exercise. Am J Physiol Endocrinol Metab. 2001 Aug;281(2):E197-206

Tipton KD, Borsheim E, Wolf SE, Sanford AP, Wolfe RR Acute response of net muscle protein balance reflects 24-h balance after exercise and amino acid ingestion. Am J Physiol Endocrinol Metab. 2003 Jan;284(1):E76-89.

van Loon LJ, Saris WH, Verhagen H, Wagenmakers AJ. Plasma insulin responses after ingestion of different amino acid or protein mixtures with carbohydrate. Am J Clin Nutr. 2000 Jul;72(1):96-105.

Myth 4. Glutamine is the Most Abundant Amino Acid in Muscle.

This is certainly one of the most explosive myths in supplement history, the misunderstanding of this concept alone has sold literally tons of product. A paradoxical myth, it conjures up the idea that glutamine is the amino acid central to building and repairing muscle. In fact, it is common to hear people refer to this myth as their sole justification for glutamine supplementation. The problem lies in the wording of the myth; that being the fact that glutamine is the most abundant amino acid <u>in</u> muscle.

Another Brick in the Wall

In order to explain properly, we must again imagine a muscle cell like a brick house. Going back to the "amino acids are bricks" analogy, we know that the 20 amino acids comprise the walls of the house. Now in order to get the muscle bigger and stronger, we need to make bigger walls by adding more bricks, which is analogous to protein synthesis. Remember that adding these amino acid bricks <u>to the walls</u> not only enlarges the muscle cell, but it also contributes to the process of muscle contraction (i.e. muscle strength).

Now it stands to reason that if glutamine is the most abundant "brick", then we need the most of this amino acid to build our muscle. The problem is that glutamine contributes very little at all to the actual walls. In fact, <u>of the 20 amino acids that we use to build our muscle, glutamine has the fourth lowest concentration</u>. Rather than being the most abundant, glutamine actually ranks 16th in abundance.

Floating Inside

So how is it that glutamine the most abundant amino acid? The answer is simply that it doesn't contribute much to the structure of muscle, but it sits *inside* the muscle cell. This is like taking our empty house and throwing a pile of glutamine bricks inside. It doesn't actually contribute to the structure of the house -which for us means that it doesn't contribute to muscle size or strength.

A decade ago it was theorized that by having more glutamine in the muscle cell could stimulate an overall anabolic effect. Although this was a good test-tube theory, it has been shown to be invalid when finally tested. In fact, consuming additional glutamine doesn't even increase the glutamine inside the cell, let alone produce an anabolic stimulus. This is expanded upon in the review on glutamine (under Supplement Reviews) as well as in the very next myth.

Quick Tip: If you like glutamine then just use it. It's really not a big deal.

Myth 5. Creatine Is the Most Anabolic Supplement

Creatine is certainly the greatest performance-enhancing supplement in history, although one of its effects is a little overplayed. The idea that creatine supplementation directly increases muscle growth has been a strong selling point, although it's not entirely accurate. This concept lies in what's known as the cellular hydration theory, and is based on the idea that filling up our cells with water will signal them to stimulate muscle growth.

More specifically, this myth consists of two parts: 1) The most important is the idea that the initial weight gain is actual, protein-based, muscle growth.
2) The second involves the exaggeration with which the cell swelling stimulates protein synthesis.

Anabolic Water

Let's back up a second and reiterate that muscle cells (like all cells) are mostly water. It often helps to imagine them as a balloon filled with water. Now the amount of water in a cell can vary depending not only on how much water we have in our body, but also how much food. The reason for the former is obvious, but food intake affects our muscle cell volume because carbohydrates and creatine (which is both naturally produced and consumed from meat) are stored inside our muscle along with *a lot* of water.

Carbohydrate and creatine molecules have a natural attraction to water, so as they are stored in muscle, they bring along a lot of water with them. Additionally, there is an 'osmotic pull' which basically means that water is pulled into the cell to keep the *ratio* of water to creatine the same -more creatine in muscle means more water is pulled in to balance out the ratio. Although this is an interesting point, it really goes beyond the scope of this discussion, so here's the punchline:

Lots of Food → Cell Swelling

Creatine: The *Real* Weight Gainer

This is why we gain so much weight when we begin to use creatine. Although it looks and feels like protein-based muscle, it is just water inside our cells. This is analogous to filling up a water balloon with more water; it still looks and feels like a balloon, it's just bigger.

That is not to say that this weight gain should be perceived as fake, it simply isn't what it appears to be. It may still serve a positive function for most people, but it isn't active contracting tissue. It does raise the point however that this weight gain may be a detriment to those who are involved in sports where minimizing weight is an issue.

Anabolic Application

So now that you know what happens, let's see how protein synthesis ties into this. If you remember from the earlier explanation about the energy requirements for protein synthesis, it takes a lot of food energy for this process to occur. Now the only time that our body has very full muscle cells is when it's well-fed. Do you see where this is going?

Cell Swelling → Permission to Turn on Protein Synthesis

Evolutionarily speaking, our cells can equate this swollen state with plenty of food, which means that it can turn on protein synthesis without fear of starvation (which is always the main concern for our body).

Lots of Food → Cell Swelling → Increased Muscle Growth

It is this elegant theory, which can be seen on cells in a test tube, that has been put forth as the reason for why creatine supplementation is anabolic. Unfortunately, when tested in healthy creatine-supplemented humans the theory almost seems to fall apart. In fact, of four such groups studied only one has shown any positive effect (and that result was slightly reduced muscle breakdown).

Practical Application

The studies in question weren't perfect and the results should always be questioned. Most importantly for us, we must ask whether the results are universally applicable, because the protein synthesis measurements were performed shortly after exercise. It is possible that creatine (a.k.a. cellular hydration) could enhance anabolism at a time other than when measured.
In fact, other studies have shown that creatine helps to promote the cell signaling to induce muscle growth, although the realistic impact of this finding is unknown.

Creatine greatly assists with muscle growth and performance, whether it is slightly anticatabolic or simply allows us to train harder. But the idea that it is super anabolic due to the observable muscle swelling and weight gain needs to die.

Selected References

Louis M, Poortmans JR, Francaux M, Berre J, Boisseau N, Brassine E, Cuthbertson DJ, Smith K, Babraj JA, Waddell T, Rennie MJ. No effect of creatine supplementation on human myofibrillar and sarcoplasmic protein synthesis after resistance exercise. Am J Physiol Endocrinol Metab. 2003 Nov;285(5):E1089-94.

Louis M, Poortmans JR, Francaux M, Hultman E, Berre J, Boisseau N, Young VR, Smith K, Meier-Augenstein W, Babraj JA, Waddell T, Rennie MJ. Creatine supplementation has no effect on human muscle protein turnover at rest in the postabsorptive or fed states.
Am J Physiol Endocrinol Metab. 2003 Apr;284(4):E764-70.

Parise G, Mihic S, MacLennan D, Yarasheski KE, Tarnopolsky MA. Effects of acute creatine monohydrate supplementation on leucine kinetics and mixed-muscle protein synthesis. J Appl Physiol. 2001 Sep;91(3):1041-7.

Willoughby DS, Rosene J. Effects of oral creatine and resistance training on myosin heavy chain expression. Med Sci Sports Exerc. 2001 Oct;33(10):1674-81

Willoughby DS, Rosene JM. Effects of oral creatine and resistance training on myogenic regulatory factor expression. Med Sci Sports Exerc. 2003 Jun;35(6):923-9

Myth 6. Amino Acids Are Just the Building Blocks of Protein

The most central concept of the Anabolic Index is that amino acids have the ability directly stimulate muscle growth and recovery, independent of training or hormonal status. This ability is called the Pharmaceutical Effect of amino acids, because although it is completely natural, it is a very powerful effect.

The reason that this idea is repeated here is because this is the cornerstone for the entire Anabolic Index. It is critical that we stop looking at food as simply fuel - instead, we need to look at nutrients in terms of how they can optimize our own biochemistry, which is exactly what The Anabolic Index does.

Quick Tip: Use The Anabolic Index. How's *that* for a tip?

Myth 7. Post-Workout Meals Are Anabolic Because They Optimize Our Hormonal Environment

One of the big selling points for post-workout nutrition is that it decreases cortisol levels after a workout (or prevents an increase). While this is certainly an interesting idea, there is little support for it. In fact, the commonly cited study to support this myth actually shows that of the three days tested, post-workout nutrition actually *increased* cortisol during the first day. Most other studies that have examined this phenomenon have shown no effect.

The point of discussing this myth is not to destroy an idea of little practical significance –it goes much deeper than that. The point is that despite the abundance of *direct* protein synthetic data, some people are still concerned with this inconsequential hormonal manipulation. While it is a nice idea to limit cortisol after a workout, this is greatly misdirecting our focus, in the face of direct muscle growth data.

For example, if all studies showed that post-workout meals increased cortisol would you stop using them? Of course not, because we have seen time and time again that the pharmaceutical effects of <u>amino acids cause a stimulation of muscle growth and recovery regardless of hormonal environment</u>. So even if testosterone and growth hormone levels dropped, we would still be in an anabolic state because of our food and/or supplementation.

Amino Acids >> Acute Hormonal Manipulation

Of course that is not to say that hormonal manipulation is not important at all. It is merely stating that in the face of *direct* nutritionally mediated protein synthetic data the hormonal data become irrelevant. In other words; we know that the ultimate effect is muscle growth.

Quick Tip: We have entered the age of biochemical manipulation through nutrition and the age that focused on archaic hormonal manipulation is at an end.

FAQ- Your [sic] wrong. You say that food is more important than hormones, but I know a guy who used testosterone and he's HUGE.

A. This is confusing a long-term use of exogenous (externally supplied) hormones with an acute change in our natural hormone levels. If you could increase your testosterone by 10-fold for several weeks, just as your "friend" did, then you too would see a dramatic change in body composition. But slightly bumping up natural testosterone levels for an hour (which is about as well as we can manage) doesn't seem do as much as optimizing our biochemistry through nutrition.

NINE

Nutritional Optimization

Bulking vs. Simultaneous Muscle Gain/Fat loss

"Quality, quality, quality: never waver from it, even when you don't see how you can afford to keep it up. When you compromise, you become a commodity and then you die."
-Gary Hirshberg

One of the most frequent questions asked about The Anabolic Index is how to employ its techniques while trying to lose fat and build muscle at the same time. I mean, how perfect would it be to not only get bigger and stronger, but also cut up at the same time!

At first glance this seems like the best way to an ideal body, but it's not. In attempting this combination you're asking your body to perform two contradictory processes at once, just as you would be if you tried to wake up and fall asleep at the same time.

While it is certainly possible to lose fat and build muscle at the same time, it is sub-optimal. Because The Anabolic Index is all about optimizing your diet and supplementation, the compromised results that occur with simultaneous cutting and building is not part of the plan.

A Chilling Analogy

The analogy I give to explain this is as follows: imagine that you're in charge of both the heating and energy supply of a small town in Southern Canada. Naturally, because southern Canada is so close to the Arctic Circle, it is cold all of the time (think polar bears, igloos —all that kind of thing). Since you're responsible for keeping the citizens warm by stoking the town's wood furnace (the only source of heat available), you have to manage the balance between keeping the fire going and managing the wood supply for the furnace.

If you use too much wood, in an effort to keep people very warm, the fuel supply will run out, the furnace will stop working, and everyone will freeze to death. Conversely, if you don't use enough wood in the furnace, because you're trying to preserve the wood stores, people will also freeze to death. So clearly you have a tremendous responsibility to keep everyone alive by maintaining balance.

Now if you have LOTS of wood coming in then you'll have no problem keeping a roaring fire in the furnace, and everyone happy. But if you have a dwindling wood supply, it would be absolutely moronic to burn the fire at a very high rate, because you'll burn through the precious wood too quickly.

Our Body The Furnace

Well our body isn't really all that different from the furnace in this analogy. Our wood fuel availability is represented by our Calorie (food) intake, and our metabolic rate is represented by the furnace. If we have a lot of food Calories coming in, our body senses this and cranks up our metabolism quite high – including muscle growth. If, on the other hand, we're on a Calorie restricted diet, our body "knows" that if our metabolic rate doesn't slow down, we'll run out of energy and die. This basic survival mechanism explains why Calorie-restricted diets only work for a short period of time before we're forced to return to a normal feeding pattern.

How Does This Relate to Muscle Growth?

Well to answer that question, it is critical that you understand the tremendous amount of energy that it costs to build muscle. Skeletal muscle is a highly active tissue that uses more energy than any other system we have, particularly in resistance trained individuals.

Even though the process of muscle contraction itself is considered very efficient, up to 80% of the energy used in this process is wasted as heat (now you know why you get hot when you exercise). Now of course you know that physical activity (which is basically a series of prolonged muscle contractions) uses a large amount of energy. In fact, many of you exercise for this very reason!

What's really interesting is that this intentionally active energy use doesn't account for the majority of time when we're not contracting muscle. Even when "resting", our muscles remain in an active, energy using, state. This is the reason why resistance training is advocated, in addition to cardio, for fat loss –we can burn Calories all of the time.

Great. Now Seriously, How Does This Relate To Muscle Growth?

What I've tried to demonstrate is that once it's built, skeletal muscle uses **a lot** of energy –a fact about which our bodies are acutely aware. But as *you're* probably aware, I haven't even addressed the actual process of *building* the muscle yet.

It shouldn't surprise you to know that the actual process of building muscle *also* takes a tremendous amount of energy. This is because we're essentially building new tissue, but only after we've gone through the process of removing all of the damaged tissue. Although it may not seem like much, that's a lot of things going on simply from throwing around a few weights.

So to reiterate, muscle growth requires a tremendous amount of energy for:

1) The actual growth
2) The maintenance of the muscle mass

Going back to our wood furnace analogy, muscle growth would equate to stoking the furnace such that it is roaring hot, and subsequently using tons of wood energy. Again, this is because of the huge energy cost of the muscle itself. Now if we're on a Calorically restricted diet, which equates to having a *low* wood supply, our body would be absolutely crazy to stoke up the fire that high (i.e. building muscle), because we're liable to run out of energy and die! So our body fights to preserve its energy supply, and one of the ways in which it does so is to limit the growth, or even reduce the amount, of this energy consuming tissue: muscle.

From Stop To Grow

In order to optimize the amount of muscle growth and recovery using the Anabolic Index, one must consume an enormous amount of Calories, such that our body knows that the energy supply (a.k.a. wood supply) is plentiful, and it's "all systems go" for growth and recovery.

We actually have a chemical "switch" if you will, that can turn on and off growth. This switch acts as a sensor or thermostat in that it senses the amount of energy in a particular cell (each cell has its own set of switches). As mentioned earlier, when the amount of energy in the cell is too low, the switch is turned off for all anabolic processes, including not only muscle recovery, but also glycogen storage. If we have plenty of energy then the switch is turned on, and muscle recovery proceeds.

Practical Application

The key is to figure out how to keep the switch in the "ON" position so we can optimize our muscle growth and recovery. After all, if this switch is off for long periods of time, this means that we're having delayed recovery at both a protein and a carbohydrate level.

The first trick to keeping the switch turned on is to ensure that we have adequate energy coming in, in the form of food. Revisiting the furnace analogy, this convinces our body that we're not going to starve so it's okay to turn up the furnace, and that all systems are GO for anabolism. This is touched upon in the "Overfeeding" section of the other manual.

Another trick to optimize recovery is to ensure that we consume enough carbohydrates <u>at the right times</u> to optimize our glycogen replenishment. This elevated level of glycogen in our cells is a sign that we have plenty of energy and keeps the switch in the ON potion.

Later in this manual, you'll learn about proper carbohydrate management, and how to utilize it to your best metabolic advantage.

Quick Tip: Pay attention to Calories! Although it's actually possible to build muscle on a hypocaloric diet, it is clearly sub optimal. Sadly the Caloric restriction isn't always intentional, as many people inadvertently starve themselves when trying to build muscle.

Selected References

Carling D. AMP-activated protein kinase: balancing the scales. Biochimie. 2005 Jan;87(1):87-91

Hue L, Rider MH. The AMP-activated protein kinase: more than an energy sensor. Essays Biochem. 2007;43:121-38

Kahn BB, Alquier T, Carling D & Hardie DG (2005). AMP-activated protein kinase: ancient energy gauge provides clues to modern understanding of metabolism. Cell Metab 1, 15–25

Sebastian B. Jørgensen, Erik A. Richter and Jørgen F. P. Wojtaszewski. Role of AMPK in skeletal muscle metabolic regulation and adaptation in relation to exercise J Physiol 574.1 pp 17-31

Wojtaszewski JF, MacDonald C, Nielsen JN, Hellsten Y, Hardie GD, Kemp BE, Kiens B & Richter EA (2003). Regulation of 5'AMP-activated protein kinase activity and substrate utilization in exercising human skeletal muscle. Am J Physiol Endocrinol Metab 284, E813–E822.

Carbohydrates: Quality, Quantity, and Timing

A somewhat enigmatic nutrient compared to the others, carbohydrate intake is important for optimizing anabolism, recovery, and performance. Acting as a double-edged sword however, carbohydrate intake must be varied depending on one's tolerance to this nutrient, as well as one's sensitivity to the hormone insulin. In doing so we will maximize anabolism and overall body composition.

Although insulin sensitivity is far more commonly used to describe the body's reaction to carbohydrates, the difference between it and carbohydrate tolerance must be highlighted so that we will be able to idealize each parameter. Despite the importance of the former for anabolism, an understanding, and subsequent application of each, is essential for optimal results.

Carbohydrate Tolerance

This often ignored parameter refers to the way in which our body (generally muscle) absorbs ingested carbohydrates; are they sucked up by muscle or stored as bodyfat? In many situations muscle carbohydrate absorption should ideally occur without much insulin release. It is only after carbohydrate tolerance is saturated that insulin becomes a factor.

Strictly speaking, rather than a definitive threshold or saturation point, there is a continuum through which our body responds -although for our purposes, thinking of a threshold is easiest. By understanding where our body's response lies on this continuum, complete with a theoretical saturation point, we'll be better able to optimize our performance, recovery, and body composition.

Insulin Sensitivity

Although similar to carbohydrate tolerance, insulin sensitivity refers to a tissue-specific responsiveness to the hormone insulin. Ideally we would like a high muscle insulin sensitivity, such that nutrients are transported more efficiently, and a low sensitivity in fat cells, which would result in less bodyfat acquisition.

In the past this idea has often been used interchangeably with carbohydrate tolerance, in spite of their fundamental differences. In order to further illustrate, let's imagine that our fight for optimal body composition and performance is like a war. In this case, carbohydrate tolerance would be the front line defense, while insulin sensitivity is the reserves. Only after carbohydrate tolerance is overwhelmed (i.e. saturated) does insulin sensitivity become predominant.

The Importance of Carbohydrate Tolerance

We place so much emphasis on the way in which our body responds to carbohydrate ingestion because this is a major determining factor for both recovery (good) and body fat acquisition (bad).

On the positive side we need to have enough carbs to optimally stimulate anabolism and restore muscle glycogen levels -and for those who have an incredibly fast oxidative metabolism (i.e. hardgainers) carbohydrate rich foods are preferable for increasing Caloric intake.

The other side of the coin is that if our carb intake is too high, we will quickly reach carbohydrate saturation, stimulate more insulin release than is needed, and bodyfat will accrue. This is like overfilling a bucket with water; a little spillover isn't a big deal, because our insulin sensitivity can mop it up. But greatly overflowing the bucket can be disastrous for body composition, as insulin sensitivity is also overwhelmed, subsequently leading to body fat gain.

Fortunately, this is easily avoided if we develop an awareness of our own carbohydrate tolerance and insulin sensitivity, and stay within reasonable limits.

Anabolic Insulin Sensitivity

Insulin sensitivity is more directly applicable to anabolism, because it does not always pertain to carbs. In fact, insulin sensitivity affects the way in which amino acids are taken up by the muscle. Since this is a primary determinant of actual muscle growth, any enhancement in this parameter is of great concern for us.

More specifically, it is most likely that the enhanced responsiveness to insulin following a workout (a.k.a. Protein Sensitivity) plays a major role in our superior anabolism during this time. This is due to the increase in building materials from enhanced transport, along with the greater demand that is induced by training.

In summary, improved insulin sensitivity may result in improved amino acid transport into muscle, which is an incredibly anabolic adaptation.

Tolerance and Sensitivity: Determining Factors

The most important determining variable of one's carbohydrate saturation point is absolute quantity of carbohydrate ingested. This in turn should change based on: natural muscle carbohydrate tolerance, general activity level, proportion of carbohydrate Calories in the diet, along with frequency, intensity, type, and duration of workout.

Insulin sensitivity changes based on the same factors, which is why the line between it and carbohydrate tolerance has been blurred for so long. Although it is important to keep the differences in mind, particularly with regard to anabolism, you will be able to see how the terms can be used interchangeably.

1) Natural Tolerance and Sensitivity

This refers to the way in which our body's naturally respond to ingested carbohydrates. If they are quickly absorbed by muscle and other non-fat tissues, then one is said to have a high natural sensitivity —and this is quite desirable. In contrast, poor carbohydrate tolerance suggests that a great deal of insulin needs to be released, which increases the likelihood of fat gain.

Natural sensitivity is dependent on a number of factors, particularly age. The older one gets, the greater the decline in insulin sensitivity and the less desirable the response.

Body fat percentage is another major determinant of natural insulin sensitivity, with leaner individuals having better sensitivity than those with more fat tissue (somewhat ironically).

The above represent the most easily determined and influential factors determining insulin sensitivity, and carbohydrate consumption should be based upon them. For example an individual who is in their 40's and can no longer be considered "lean" should use fewer carbohydrates due to a likelihood of diminished insulin sensitivity.

Quick Tip: The Sleep Test

One good measure of your insulin sensitivity is to pay attention to how you feel after consuming a non-workout related carb source. If you feel sleepy within half an hour of the meal, it could represent poor insulin sensitivity. By paying attention to the entire content of the meal (including fats and proteins) you will eventually be able to see a pattern develop of which foods make you sleepy —ideally it should be none. Although this isn't a sure fire way of determining insulin sensitivity, it can be a powerful tool in determining how many grams of carbs to have in each meal.

2) General Activity Level

This one is simple because the more active an individual is the greater the insulin sensitivity they will have. This means that a greater number of carbohydrates can be tolerated by the body, and are likely required for optimal performance. This does not specifically refer to spiking blood sugar levels after a workout, but simply the overall number of carbohydrates consumed throughout the day.

Key Point: As a general rule, glycogen depletion will be the determining factor for overall carbohydrate quantity.

Age/Activity Level/Bodyfat % $\Rightarrow$ Long Term Insulin Sensitivity $\Rightarrow$ Long Term Carb Needs

3) Type of Workout

As more of an acute measure, this factor will mostly affect short-term carbohydrate tolerance and subsequent carbohydrate feeding.

For many people the type of workout is just the difference between training legs or arms, while for others it consists of going for a 2 hour run while adding in Fartlek training (general athletic activity that makes use of the surrounding environment e.g. chin-ups on a tree branch) along the way. These extremes represent completely different levels of carbohydrate depletion, and subsequently require different recommendations for carbohydrate intake.

Training Type/Intensity $\Rightarrow$ Glycogen Depletion $\Rightarrow$ Acute Carb Tolerance $\Rightarrow$ Short Term Carb Needs

Resistance Training

Contrary to popular belief, resistance training uses up relatively little muscle glycogen, when compared to other forms of exercise. This quantity is even further reduced by a lower rep range and heavier weights. Perhaps a more important consideration is the amount of muscle mass worked during the session. A leg workout will more significantly deplete endogenous carbohydrate stores, while an arm or shoulder workout will have little impact. By keeping this in mind we can tailor our carbohydrate intake to meet the depletion needs.

Other Types of Training

Activity involving a significant aerobic component can greatly deplete muscle and whole body glycogen stores such that a large replenishment is required. Whether it is a 2-hour football practice or hitting the treadmill for an hour, glycogen stores will be depleted to a much greater extent than with resistance training alone.

Key Point: It is critical to note that these recommendations are for use with the intention of optimizing lean muscle growth and maximal recovery. Carbohydrate intake regulations during a diet directed toward fat loss would be far more strict, while those geared toward maximizing aerobic endurance performance might be more liberal.

Practical Application: Timing

Using the aforementioned criteria as a guide, we will be able to determine the limits of our carbohydrate tolerance and stay within them. The next important step is to figure out when the carbohydrates should be consumed.

Note: Post-workout/acute carbohydrate ingestion guidelines are discussed in the "Post-Workout Nutrition" section.

Morning

It is optimal for lean muscle gain if the majority of carbohydrates are consumed earlier in the day. This is due to a progressive impairment in carbohydrate tolerance as the day progresses. A nighttime fast (protein fasting excepted) will reverse this trend and essentially "reset" our high Carbohydrate Tolerance for the next day.

For the first liquid meal of the day, up to a 1:1 ratio of carbohydrates: protein is warranted, although carbohydrate quantity may be altered depending on the one's tolerance.

In spite of all the immediate post-workout hype, we know that post-workout insulin sensitivity is enhanced for more than 24 hours following a training bout. This means that our carbohydrate tolerance is greatly enhanced, simply by virtue of training. Although this effect significantly affects the quantity of carbohydrates that we may consume without deleterious effect, it is still recommended that the guide below be used to determine overall intake.

Quantity Guidelines for Carbohydrate Tolerance

High: carbohydrate intake as needed, but greatly reduced or absent in the final pre-sleep meal.

Moderate: 2/3 of carbs ingested throughout the first half of the day, and tapered down as the day progresses. Carbohydrates may be used with one or two Protein Pulse Feedings, ideally pre-workout.

Low: carbohydrate consumption is divided exclusively between the waking meal and the hour following a workout (overall quantity is kept low). No carbohydrates are used with Protein Pulse Feeding.

Practical Application: Quality

For the most part, carbohydrate quality is kept as high as possible throughout the day. This means that the types of carbohydrates ingested should consist of those that are digested relatively slowly. This will ensure a moderate insulin release, at most, which will help to minimize both fat gain and induction of sleepiness. Consuming the majority of carbohydrates with vegetables and fats also helps to ensure that Protein is Protected (**Key #5**) and acute insulin levels are kept low.

The main exceptions for carbohydrate quality are during Protein Pulse Feeding, and pre/post-workout. During these times it is desirable to consume rapidly absorbed carbohydrates, which aids with the anabolic response. This point is expanded upon throughout the manual.

Fats And Fiction

No nutrition manual would be complete without a discussion of fats. Rather than a redundant explanation of what fats are, a more applicable description of how they can work for us is warranted.

Fats Are Bad For You

The heading embodies thinking from more than two decades ago, and still seems to have a strangle hold on the general populace. Let me say it here, once and for all that not all fats are bad, and even most of those that are, aren't bad all of the time. In fact, many fats have positive effects on our health and can be used to not only improve this parameter, but also anabolism and performance.

Much the same way that proteins have different amino acid composition and structure, fats too vary slightly in the way that they form —and can have dramatically different effects on our body.

How Fats Work For Us

For our purposes, the main effect of fats stems from their incorporation into our cell membranes. This means that the fats we eat actually become part of the biological "bags" or "casing" that surrounds our cells. But far from inert areas, these bags are a living fluid environment that have a predominant role in the way our cells work. What's important for us to know is that it is the composition of fat in our diet that affects the fats in our cell membranes, and many subsequently biochemical effects (not the least of which involve muscle growth and fat loss).

For example, we might recognize that certain hormones (such as insulin) bind to receptors on the outside of our cells. These receptors are actually part of the cell membrane and can be greatly affected by the membrane itself. Depending on the types of fats, and the quantities of each, in our cell membranes, we can improve or inhibit the way in which the receptor works.

Inflammatory Remarks

Another important example involves the way in which our cells (including muscle) respond to stress, such as exercise. Again, the type of fats in our cell membranes, and the quantity of each, will play a critical role in how that cell, and ultimately the whole body, reacts. This is particularly true for the process of inflammation, which results from any form of cellular stress. The muscle damage that we induce from training is no exception in that it triggers an inflammation response.

Without getting into detail, inflammation is a series of chemical reactions occurring in our cells, and it all starts with -you guessed it- the type and quantity of fats in our cell membranes. Some of you may even recognize that by consuming fish oil, we can increase the amount of Omega-3 fats in our cell membranes, and subsequently reduce the inflammation response. More specifically, this effect is known to have both anticatabolic and antianabolic properties to muscle.

It is this keystone placement of fats in the cell membrane that make them such a powerful mediator of inflammation and subsequent responses –they are at the beginning of the reaction, while other antiinflammatories tend to deal with the ensuing chemical reactions.

Other Effects

Naturally this brief discussion of fats only scratches the surface of how fats work, but it is critical to understand that when we ingest them, they become part of our body and have a tremendous impact on our biochemistry.

In summary, muscle building effects include: hormone production (for muscle growth and fat loss), adaptability of nerve cells -including our brain- (for muscle strength), faster recovery, decreased muscle breakdown, and improved hormonal responsiveness.

Types of Fat

Along with the understanding of the effects of fats, it is important to consider the individual types of fat and their sources.

1) Omega-3

For its health benefits, this is the best type of fat we can consume. Unfortunately, along with its effectiveness comes an instability (e.g. light and temperature sensitivity) that requires special care when purchasing and consuming. High levels of these fats are found in flax, walnuts, fish, and their respective oils. Highly recommended.

2) Omega-6

Now the predominant type of fat in our diet, omega-6 fats come from natural sources such as corn, safflower, and sunflower oils. Although they are moderately healthy compared to most fats, most people over consume them at the expense of omega-3's. Decreased intake is usually warranted.

3) Monounsaturated

Olive oil is considered the main monounsaturated fat, and has a host of healthy benefits to go along with it. Considered the main cooking oil, the benefits of olive oil are apparent in the popularity of the Mediterranean diet. Other sources include avocados and canola oil, along with almonds, cashews, and macadamia nuts. Highly recommended.

4) Saturated

So named due to the chemical structure, saturated fat is the predominant type in most animal products. Although not inherently harmful, people grossly over consume saturated fat and unfortunately must contend with the resulting health problems. Complete omission of this fat is not warranted, although a decreased intake usually is.

5) Trans

It seems as though trans fats (a.k.a. Hydrogenated oils) are being recognized as public enemy number one, and this is a good thing indeed. Trans fats are chemically altered natural fats —warped such that they are more "user friendly" and resist going bad. Due to the negative health implication of consuming these fats, complete bans on their use are now occurring. In spite of their prevalence in our society, this type of fat has no place in anyone's diet.

Practical Application

Fats are best consumed with any meal that is not meant to involve Protein Pulse Feeding. Acutely, they help to stabilize blood sugar and add satiety to any meal. Overall quantity is dependent on both Carbohydrate Tolerance and overall Caloric requirements.

For example, the lower one's carbohydrate tolerance, the more fat is warranted in the diet, at the expense of both carbohydrates and Calories. Alternatively, if one has little appetite, but a high carbohydrate tolerance, then fats may be used as needed to supplement Calories. Due to their high Caloric density compared to other nutrients, fats work well in this regard —too well for most people.

Percentages of Percentages

As far as percentage of one's diet, fats usually make up 33-50% when trying to increase lean muscle mass. Again, the specifics of this percentage are refined based on Caloric requirements, carbohydrate tolerance, and personal preference.

The derivation of fats should also be of concern, due to the differing effect of each type. For the majority of people, a ratio of 1:1:1:1 (Omega-3: Omega-6: Monounsaturated: Saturated) is most effective. Note that trans fats are completely eliminated.

For a quick and dirty example, we can use the usual 200lb heavy training athlete. If he needs 4000 Calories a day for lean muscle growth, then 2000 Calories, or approximately 200g, of fat is optimal. This works out nicely between 50g of each type of fat.

Quick Tip: Fatty acid incorporation into cell membranes is a lengthy process; so do not worry if exact ratios are not met each day. It is simple enough to make up for it with subsequent meals. For example, if you miss out on monounsaturated fats one day, simply have more in the following day or two.

Meal Timing: A 21st Century Approach

In trying to optimize our internal biochemistry, and subsequently our results, then it is important to consider meal timing in a global sense. While this aspect is widely considered in the time surrounding our workout, it is equally important to consider other times as well.

Employing The Dogma

The first point that needs to be addressed is that of the 3-hour rule. This states that if you eat every three hours then you will have both increased muscle growth and fat loss. There are three main ideas behind this:

1) Anabolic Stream: by providing a continuous stream of protein for our muscle, we will be able to optimize growth.

2) Insulin Maintenance: by maintaining a steady intake of food, we are able to stabilize insulin levels, and subsequently minimize bodyfat acquisition.

3) Metabolic Boost: by ensuring that our body will never enter a "starvation mode", our metabolic rate is not turned down for the sake of self-preservation (which happens whenever we are lacking cellular energy). This means that our metabolic rate will remain high at all times.

For someone who has never considered anything other than eating when hungry, or "three square meals a day", this novel concept may seem earth shattering. But we have to ask ourselves: is it optimal?

While there is nothing inherently harmful about eating every few hours, it seems to have been taken to an extreme by many people –to the point of being dogmatic. But what are they basing it on? Could we actually be hurting our progress from this? Yes.

Hindering Anabolism

Let's first examine the idea that a steady influx of amino acids is ideal for growth. Clearly based on what we know about Protein Pulse Feeding and protein resistance, an amino acid flatline is exactly the *opposite* of what we want! Recall that our body responds to increasing levels of amino acids in the bloodstream, while a flatline represents the death of muscle growth.

It is inevitable that we'll have a steady influx of amino acids into our bloodstream, because it is impractical to Protein Pulse all day, we should not be fooled into thinking that such a practice is optimal.

Quick Tip: Recent preliminary research suggests that eating several small meals a day (to maintain a steady amino acid flow to muscle) is less effective for muscle growth than eating only a few large meals. This is likely due to the elimination of any type of protein pulse feeding. Expect to hear more about this in the future.

The Good Points

Moving on to the idea of steady insulin, this one has some evidence behind it. Outside of a morning shake, or the drinks consumed pre/post-workout, insulin it is generally ideal to keep insulin low. This not only allows us to maintain a state of fat loss, but also minimizes the amount of fat that is stored (a subtle but important distinction). One might go so far as to argue that the 3-hour rule is ideal solely based on this concept, but we have to consider what it is that we're avoiding if we time our meals differently.

Going To Extremes

Let's pretend for a minute that insulin management and metabolic maintenance are ideal when we eat every few hours. Based on this, we need to explore what would happen if we eat more or less frequently. For example, if we have a large steak meal complete with salad (and oil dressing), and chocolate cake for dessert. Do we need to eat again 3 hours later, even if we're still feeling full? Of course not! This is but the first problem with the 3-hour generalization.

On the other extreme, if we have a waking protein shake that consists of whey hydrolysate and glucose; should we wait for 3 hours before feeding? Of course not! Not only would we be protein fasted for a couple of hours (which we know from **Key # 3**, and the review of whey protein, is especially catabolic), and we may even experience a blood sugar crash (which is also quite catabolic –not to mention unpleasant).

The Key Is Feeding

When we think of feeding, we of course think of food going into our mouths. While this makes practical sense for every day living, it is not the way our cells experience feeding –and it is what our cells experience that is critical for optimization.

Recall that once our food enters the gut, it has to be digested and then absorbed. The nutrients then enter the bloodstream, from which they enter the cells. It is imperative to really think about this, because when we do, it becomes clear that our cells are fed from our gut, not the mouth. This in turn means that the 3-hour rule is not universally optimal because it does not take into account how the body is actually fed!

Why We Feed

If we're focusing on our cells being fed from the gut and bloodstream, then this will change the way in which we feed from the mouth, at least temporally. Let's go back to the extreme examples to illustrate how this should work in practice.

1) The Slow Meal

If we're eating a large meal replete with fat and slow digesting protein, then it is clear that our body will be fed for many hours to come. This is because the fat, and slow protein (and possibly the fiber) will induce a slow digestion/absorption of nutrients, which will provide our cells with a steady influx of nutrients. Consuming more food, three hours later (for example), would create a backlog in our gut, which is still full from the previous meal. This can have a negative impact on digestion as well as contribute to Caloric excess (which at the very least is suboptimally carried out here), and potential digestive upset.

2) The Fast Meal

Consuming a fast digesting/absorbing drink in the morning will result in a rapid protein, and possibly insulin, pulse. This is optimal for anabolism and recovery, but care must be taken to feed again shortly thereafter. The reason is because everything is absorbed so quickly that there may actually be a deficit once the nutrients are used! This means that our internal anabolic environment can quickly become catabolic if care is not taken. Not to worry, because simply consuming more food (or another drink) 60 minutes after the fast shake will satisfy all requirements.

Practical Application

Now that we understand the importance of meal timing, it is critical to figure out the "How To's". Initially this takes a bit of attention to the type of foods we eat and how our body reacts. For example, if we eat a meal and become hot from it (a natural phenomenon known as Diet Induced Thermogenesis a.k.a. DIT), then it means that our body is still dealing with the food and we don't need to feed again. Of course it is important to distinguish this body temperature variation from that induced by exercise or environmental factors.

We can also measure how our body responds to carbohydrate containing meals by the amount of fatigue or sleepiness they can induce. For example, if you eat a large meal and become sleepy after it, this means that you've had a large insulin response to the meal, and may need to eat again sooner than is otherwise optimal (for the sake of our blood sugar maintenance).

Quick Tip: People often attribute post-meal sleepiness to the amino acid tryptophan. While it is involved, the sedative effect is more practically attributable to a large release of insulin. After all, our high protein diets are replete with tryptophan, but not every meal induces the sedative effect. By paying attention to this variable, you will be able to determine how your body responds to particular meals, and adjust future meal timing accordingly.

Conclusion

It may take a little bit of work to determine how your body responds to certain foods and their combinations, but the results will be worth it. While we have to work within the practical limits of our lifestyle, it is possible to eat based on optimal temporal parameters, and eat "normally" as well. They are not mutually exclusive concepts. Most importantly, the effect on our body composition, performance, and even health will be dramatic.

Putting It All Together

There is a tremendous amount of new data in this manual, so this section is required such that we can see how it all works as a whole. Think of it like putting the individual pieces of a puzzle together to yield the optimal result.

NOTE: See "Of Masses and Measures" section for common unit conversions and protein quantities of common foods.

In the following examples, we will use a lean (10% bodyfat) and active 220lb (100kg) athlete.

Getting Started: Step 1

The first thing we need to figure out is how many Calories we need each day. This can be done by using the multiplier as discussed below.

Example:

220lb individual with 10% bodyfat =200lbs lean mass

NOTE: Estimates of bodyfat percentage are fine for a starting point.

Caloric estimates are paired with a specific multiplier depending on several individual factors.

Multiplier: This number ranges from 10-20 and is used to determine an initial Caloric target when combined with the quantity of lean body mass.

Considerations for choosing a multiplier: There are numerous factors that will affect the choice of a multiplier. Some examples include: activity level, natural metabolic rate, level of muscle mass, and body fat percentage.

Example: Considering that our hypothetical subject is quite active and has a moderate level of lean body mass 18 is chosen as a starting multiplier. As always, this number will be adjusted depending on how he responds to the diet.

200lbs x 18= 3600 Calories a day

For someone who is less active, multiplying by a lower number is warranted – only you know how active you are, and how your own body will respond to a high Calorie intake. Of course we're using rough numbers, but it has been my experience with clients that these are great starting points. From there, we will refine Caloric requirements based on results. Such fluidity and evolution is the only way to truly personalize your program.

Macronutrient Breakdown: Step 2

Next, we need to figure out our macronutrient breakdown, within the realistic limits of our Caloric requirements. This also has the luxury of being based on lifestyle and personal preferences, with carbohydrate tolerance acting as a major determining factor.

Example: Our subject is moderately lean and trains hard and frequently, so he will have a greater carbohydrate tolerance. Fortunately, he has a taste for carbs, which will help him meet his Caloric needs (which can often be a struggle).

Macronutrient proportions are determined before actual quantity, and as you might expect, it all hinges on protein. Daily protein quantity is determined by the calculation of lean body mass x 1.5g.

$$200\text{lbs} \times 1.5 = 300\text{g protein daily}$$

Carbohydrates and fats will make up equal parts of the diet (Calorically speaking), which can now be calculated. Using this information, along with the appropriate Caloric mass conversion (i.e. Carbohydrates and Protein yield 4 Calories per gram, and Fat yields 9 Calories per gram), the breakdown would be as follows:

$$300\text{g Protein} \times 4 = 1200 \text{ Calories}$$

3600 (total Calories) – 1200 (protein Calories) = 2400 Calories (divided evenly between carbohydrates and fat)

$$300\text{g Carbohydrates} \times 4 = 1200 \text{ Calories}$$
$$133\text{g Fat} \times 9 = 1200 \text{ Calories}$$

or if you prefer: 33:33:33 (P:C:F)

NOTE: It should be emphasized that the isocaloric proportion is simply a coincidence in this case.

Quick Reminder: It is important to remember that your numbers are simply a guide, and will easily vary from day to day. This is fine as long as it all averages out, more or less, every 4 days.

Meal Distribution: Step 3

Now we know how much of everything we're supposed to be eating, but how does it fit into our diet? If we divide the quantities of each nutrient by 5 meals a day (for example), then we come up with an overly simplistic and impractical plan. Instead, it is best to work out your meal times and go from there.

Example:

7:00 AM Morning Shake (1)
8:30 Meal (2)
1:00 PM Meal (3)
5:00 Pre-Workout Meal (4)
6:30 Post-Workout Meal (5)
7:15 Meal (6)
11:00 Pre-Bed Meal (7)

Remember that this is only an example. It is not a suggestion that you actually eat 7 meals a day (even though this was a workout day).

Key Point: Note that meal timing is dependent on meal type and lifestyle, which is consistent with "Meal Timing: A 21st Century Approach".

Temporal Nutrient Distribution: Step 4

Once we have the meal times established by our work/school/lifestyle schedule, we need to get an approximate nutrient distribution for each meal. While it is easy to come pretty close with liquid meals, solid meals are a little more difficult.

If we start with the liquid meals for this day, we can eliminate half of the meals and end up with a more precise nutrient distribution.

From the other sections, we know that the first meal will be approximately 40P/30C/0F (grams of protein, carbohydrates, and fats, respectively). The pre and post-workout meals will be averaged to 45P/30C/0F, and the final meal of the day will be 60P/0C/35F. This eliminates a total of 190P/90C/35F, or 1435 Calories a day.

From here we can evenly (give or take) distribute the rest of the nutrient requirements across the remaining 3 meals, or 110P/210C/98F ÷ 3.

NOTE: Carbohydrate quantity is generally higher in solid meals due to the slowed digestion (and subsequent reduction of insulin).

Reminder: Keep in mind that a *range* of nutrient values are trying to be met, rather than actually matching an exact number (e.g. "I must eat 30g of protein, 80g of carbs, and 30g of fat in this meal").

Example:

Meal	P	C	F
7:00 AM Morning Shake	40g	30	0
8:30 Meal 2	30g	80	10
1:00PM Meal 3	25g	75	40
5:00 Pre-Workout Meal	40g	30	0
6:30 Post Workout Meal	50g	30	0
7:15 Meal 6	35g	45	30
11:00 Pre-Bed Meal	60g	0	35
TOTAL	280	290	115

=3315 Calories

Note that the Caloric total is a little low, and the nutrient quantities are not exact - in fact, this example is far closer to what is actually possible for most people, and that is completely acceptable. We need to work within the limits of what is *realistically* attainable.

Adding Supplements: Step 5

Supplement use is dependent on the individual, but our subject is concerned with optimal muscle growth and performance. Although money is always a limiting factor, it is not completely restrictive in this example.

7AM Morning Shake
20g Whey Hydrolysate
20g Whey Isolate
20g Sucrose
10g Glucose
10g BCAA
5g Beta Alanine
500mg Carnitine Tartrate

8:30 Meal 2

½ Multivitamin
3g EFA Oil Caps

1:00 PM Meal 3
10g BCAA

5:00 Pre-Workout Meal
30g Whey Hydrolysate
10g Whey Isolate
20g Glucose
10g Waxy Maize Starch
5g BCAA

6:30 Post Workout Meal
20g Whey Hydrolysate
30g Whey Isolate
20g Glucose
10g Waxy Maize Starch
5g BCAA
5g Creatine Monohydrate
¼ tsp Table Salt
5g Beta Alanine
500mg Carnitine Tartrate

10:15
ZMA (40mg zinc and 560mg magnesium)

11:00 Pre-Bed Meal
60g Casein
15g Flax Oil
15g Olive Oil
½ Multivitamin
10g BCAA
3g EFA Oil Caps
500mg Carnitine Tartrate

Quick Reminders

Recall that we want to keep the morning, pre and post-workout meals as quickly digestible and absorbable as possible. This is accomplished by using the ingredients listed.

The pre and post-workout meals occur 15 minutes before and after the workout, respectively.

The final meal of the day must sustain the body throughout the night. This is accomplished by using a slow digesting protein and fat, which will facilitate steady amino acid release into the bloodstream.

Quick Tips

- Multivitamin is split up to ensure a more even distribution and minimize their waste

- EFA oil caps are used with slower digesting meals only

- 60g of casein is used, instead of the recommended 80g, due to financial limitation

- Beta alanine and creatine supplementation are used post-workout to take advantage of the body's enhanced need, and assisted uptake from the other drink components

- BCAA use is spread throughout the day to maximize the effect and minimize oxidation

- Recall that table salt is used to ensure optimal creatine uptake into muscle

Concluding Remarks

This is only meant to be a good example, although it resembles an idealized program for many readers out there. By taking a stepwise approach to diet development, the otherwise complicated process is made far easier. Nutrition specifics are to be formed using the guidelines illustrated throughout the rest of this manual. Finally, only after the meal composition and timing are complete may supplements be introduced into the equation.

By putting all of this together, you will no doubt optimize your muscle growth, recovery and performance. Now go out there and get to it!

Protein Shake Recipes

No nutrition and supplementation manual would be complete without a listing of the authors' favorite protein shake recipes. Considering how important protein is to our diets, this section is critical for maintaining interest and avoiding dietary monotony.

The Mimosa-Perfect for summer days.
1/2 cup frozen mango
1/2 cup frozen peaches
1 banana
8 oz orange juice
2 tbls flax seed
40 g. vanilla protein

The Crantini-This drink is quite refreshing, and a favorite after working in the heat outside.
1/2 cup frozen raspberries
4 ice cubes
8 oz cranberry juice
8 oz raspberry yogurt
40 g protein

The Proteinaccino-Great for coffee lovers.
2 tsp instant coffee
5-6 ice cubes
12 oz milk
2 tbls heavy cream
40 g chocolate protein

Pumpkin Pie-This works well in colder weather, or it could be a nice change from more fruity drinks.
1/2 c. pumpkin puree
1 banana
8 oz vanilla yogurt
2 tbls flax seeds
dash of pumpkin pie spice
4 oz milk
2 tbls heavy cream
40 g. vanilla protein

Cherry Cheesecake-Cheesecake. Come on, what more do I need to say?
3/4 cup frozen cherries
2 graham crackers
1/2 cup vanilla yogurt
1/2 cup cottage cheese
I cup milk
2 tbls flax seeds
40 g Vanilla protein

The (not-so) Bloody Mary-A little different twist on the typical drink, this one might be an acquired taste.
16 oz V-8
2 tbls olive oil
dash of pepper
40 g unflavored protein

Key Lime Pie-Another refreshing drink, this can be made to taste by changing the juice/yogurt content.
2 oz lime juice
2 graham crackers
2 tbls walnuts
one container lime yogurt
8 oz milk
40 g vanilla protein

Peanut Butter Cookie-Who doesn't love cookies? Try this with chocolate protein powder for an even better treat.
1/3 cup peanut butter
1 banana
1/2 cup cottage cheese
1/2 cup yogurt
4 ice cubes
8 oz milk
40 g protein

Cherry-Almond Barrk-A thick great-tasting drink for a meal-like feel.
1 cup frozen cherries
1/4 cup almond butter
6 oz cherry or vanilla yogurt
8 oz oatmeal
8 oz milk
40 g protein

Of Masses and Measures

"Dear God of England, please get me out of this. If you do, I promise to spell 'color' with a U, and use the metric system with every cubic milliliter of blood in my...oh I can't do it! It's too stupid!"
-Homer Simpson

There is a lot of quantification involved in a diet and supplementation plan, and sometimes the units can get a little confusing. In order to remove all of the guesswork here is a list of all common Metric/Imperial conversions you'll need, along with some common protein serving information.

Mass:

1 Kilogram (Kg) = 1000 Grams (g)
1 Gram = 1000 Milligrams (mg)
1 Kilogram ≈ 2.2 pounds (lbs) ≈ 35.3 Ounces (oz)

Volume:

1 Litre (L) = 1000 millilitres (mL)
1 Litre ≈ 34 Fluid Ounces (fl oz.) ≈ 2 Pints ≈ 4 Cups

Cooking (U.S. and International):

1 Cup = 8 fl oz. = 16 Tablespoons (tbsp) = 48 Teaspoons
1 Tablespoon = 3 Teaspoons
1 Tablespoon = 0.5 fl oz. ≈ 15 mL

Foods and Nutrients:

Oil
1tbsp = 15g

Powdered Carbohydrates (e.g. sucrose, glucose)
1 tbsp = 12g*
* (varies with grain size)

Protein Serving Sizes

Food	Size	Protein (grams)
Milk	8 oz	8g
Chicken breast	4 oz	25g
Cottage Cheese	8 oz.	30g
Egg (whole)	1	6g
Egg (White)	1	3.5g
Egg (Yolk)	1	2.5g
Hamburger	8 oz	40g
Roast Beef	8 oz	33.5g
Sirloin Steak	7 oz	30g
Salmon	4 oz	25g
Tuna	6 oz	33g
Turkey breast	4 oz.	32g

Glossary

80-Gram Casein Protocol – the practice of consuming a large quantity of casein protein before a prolonged fast (such as sleep).

AMPK – AMP-activated protein Kinase. a.k.a. the starvation protein complex. A marker of cellular energy status. When activated, AMPK indicates that there is little energy in the cell, which in turn shuts off anabolic processes.

Accommodation Effect – a.k.a. protein resistance -a process by which our body becomes resistant to protein synthetic stimulating ability of ingested amino acids. This effect occurs when there is a steady level of amino acids in the blood.

Anabolic – an energy-consuming process of building larger molecules from smaller molecules. Colloquially refers to a substance or practice that induces muscle growth.

Anabolic Potential - The ability for something to stimulate muscle growth. A high anabolic potential is something that possesses a strong tendency to induce hypertrophy.

Carbohydrate Tolerance – the ability of muscle to absorb carbohydrates independent of the effects of insulin. A buffer zone prior to insulin release.

Cell Volumization – a.k.a. the "happy cell theory". A theory stating that the amount of water in a cell is directly related to the nutritional state, which in turn signals Anabolic processes.

Directed Placebo Effect – The perception that an inert substance is having a physical effect, which is enhanced by a preconceived notion of a specific function for that substance.

DOMS - Delayed Onset Muscle Soreness. The feeling of pain that often follows a day or two after resistance training. This transient pain is a result of the inflammation response stemming from training-induced muscle damage and may be correlated with hypertrophy.

Hypertrophy (muscle) – muscle growth.

Intermediate Speed Protein – a protein that maintains amino acids in the bloodstream for a moderate duration. Examples include such as whey isolate and whey concentrate.

Loading Supplement - a type of supplement that is initially consumed in high doses in order to maximize our cellular levels of that supplement (e.g. creatine and beta alanine). After the "loading phase" a lower, "maintenance", dose is used.

Muscle Insulin Sensitivity - the ability with which our muscle responds to the hormone insulin. A high sensitivity is desirable for muscle growth and health.

Nutrient Density - a measure of Caloric or nutrient content by volume of the food. For example, a high nutrient density food would contain a large number of Calories while being relatively small.

Oxidative Damage – cellular/molecular damage induced by free radical molecules. This can be mitigated by use of antioxidant substances, such as vitamin C.

Paradoxical Myth - a true statement that has been bastardized to the point that the meaning is practically incorrect or skewed.

Pharmaceutical Effect (of Amino Acids) – the ability of amino acids and protein to stimulate protein synthesis independent of training or hormonal status. The key concept on which the Anabolic Index is based.

Post-Workout Blackout Period - the time immediately following resistance training when the pharmaceutical effect of amino acids may be blunted. A time of protein resistance.

Post-Workout Window – an archaic notion that following resistance exercise, there is a short time in which our body is more sensitive to nutrient utilization. It is based on outdated/inapplicable science and still perpetuated by the majority of the fitness/bodybuilding industry.

Priming The Pump – using specifically timed pre-workout nutrition in order to maximize blood flow, anabolism, and the muscle pump.

Protein Resistance - a time in which our muscle is less responsive to the pharmaceutical effect of protein. This occurs during the post-workout blackout and during a flatline of amino acids in the bloodstream.

Protein Sensitivity – a state in which our muscle is more sensitive to the pharmaceutical effect of protein. The days following resistance training are the prime example of such a time.

Saturation Point – the point at which muscle becomes replete with a particular substance, such as creatine or beta-alanine. The point at which the loading phase is terminated and the maintenance phase begins.